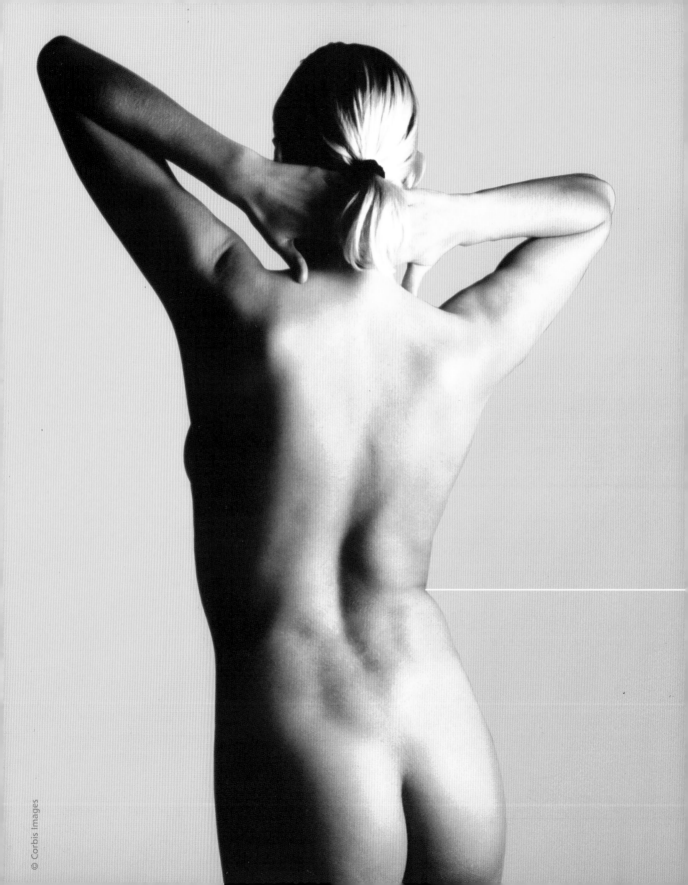

THE CELLULITE CURE™

by Dr. Lionel Bissoon

ISBN 0-9764821-0-X

PUBLISHED BY MESO PRESS
8400 Menaul NE • Suite 162 • Albuquerque, NM 87112
www.cellulitecure.com

Creative Director Leslie Fischer
Cover Design by Leslie Fischer
Cover Photograph by Steve Ladner

Illustrations and Charts by Zane Fix, Brent Hartman, M. Hurley and Thomas Penna.
Cartoons by Zane Fix.
Design, Art Direction by Teknigrammaton Graphics, Inc.
773-973-1614 • www.Teknigram.com • Teknigram@ATTGlobal.net
7312 N. Hamilton • Chicago, Illinois 60645

Color Correction by Sebastian Pineda • www.SebastianPineda.com
917-939-5907 • 108-25 72 Ave., Ste. 3e • Forest Hills, NY 11375

Photography by Dr. Lionel Bissoon, Graciela Cattarossi and Steve Ladner.
Printed in Seoul, Korea by Samhwa Printing Co., Ltd.

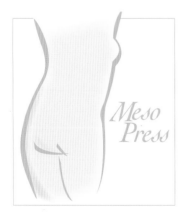

Disclaimer

The information contained in this book is based on medical literature, scientific research and professional experience. The author has extensively researched the information contained in this book; since science is constantly changing, however, there are no guarantees to its completeness.
The information provided is the most recent and up to date at the time of writing. The information provided is not a substitute for competent medical advice. The publisher and author are not responsible for any adverse reaction attributable to Mesotherapy treatments or to suggestions made in this book. All cartoon characters depicted in this book are fictions and any resemblance to any person, living or dead, is purely coincidental.

contents

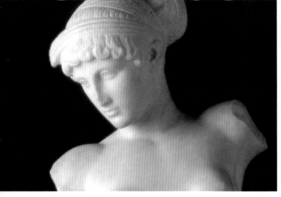

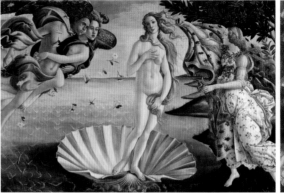

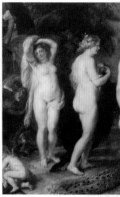

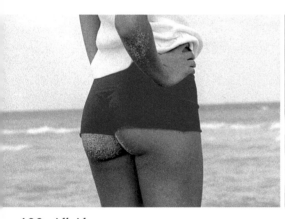

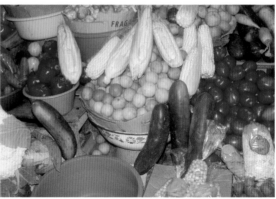

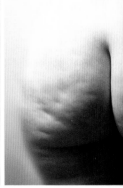

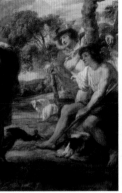
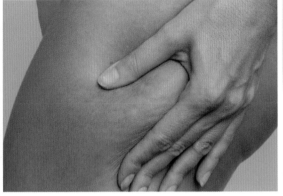
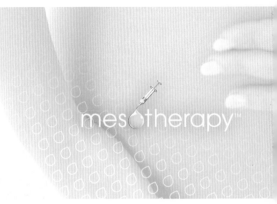

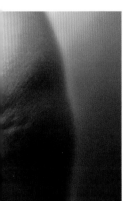
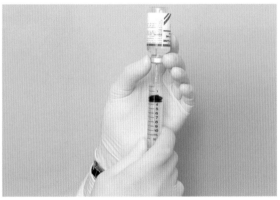
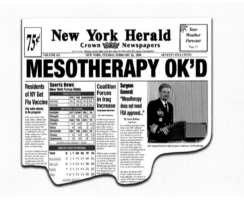

Acknowledgments

To my mom, thank you for encouraging me in all of my endeavors. You allowed me to pursue my dreams and supported me in all my wild and crazy moments. My friend Grace Trombly, thanks for the bananas, Vernon's ginger ale and the Kit-Kat candy bars. They kept me going during difficult times. But more importantly, all of your encouragement, understanding and support made a world of difference.

To my friend Dr. James X. Hartman, you cultivated, nurtured and nourished my mind. You said the question one should ask himself on a daily basis is, "Did you make a difference?" These words have been the basis of my work. Thank you.

My Creative Director and Assistant, Leslie Fischer, without your encouragement, hard work, and many late nights this book would still be in my head. Your creative insights transformed my thoughts into this book. Liz Belson, the perpetual promoter—thank you. My medical assistant Nela, who has been with me from the beginning of this Mesotherapy adventure, I appreciate all your efforts. My friends Oz Garcia and Heidi Krupp— without your efforts Mesotherapy would still be in its infancy in the U.S.A.

To my friend and patient, Roberta Flack, thank you for your generosity and willingness to tell the world about your positive experiences with Mesotherapy.

To Peter Hutt who graciously consented to be interviewed. Your contribution to Mesotherapy gives so much validity and credibility to this new specialty. Your legal guidance is a valuable asset. This work would not be possible without the valuable contribution of Peter Gerado.

To the memory of Dr. Michel Pistor, it was your dream to see Mesotherapy become accepted in the U.S.A. This book was inspired by your dream.

My friends and faculty at the Bissoon Institute of Mesotherapy, Dr. Lee Elber, Dr. Ronald Rothenberg, Dr. Denise Brunner, Dr. Frank Greenway, Dr. James Hartman, Dr. Douglas Broadfield, Dr. Tommy Guillot, Katie Caruso and Dr. Salvatore Cavalier, your dedication, support and enthusiasm is a testament to the success of Mesotherapy.

To all the patients who graciously volunteered the use of their before and after photographs for this book. This gift will empower many women who have struggled with cellulite. Thank you!

My Guru, Sri Siva you have treated me like a son and have nourished my soul. You taught me to manifest my dreams through your meditation techniques. This book is a manifestation of your student. More importantly, you have been my ray of light from the moment I met you.

Acknowledgements • VIII

Dedicated to my son William...

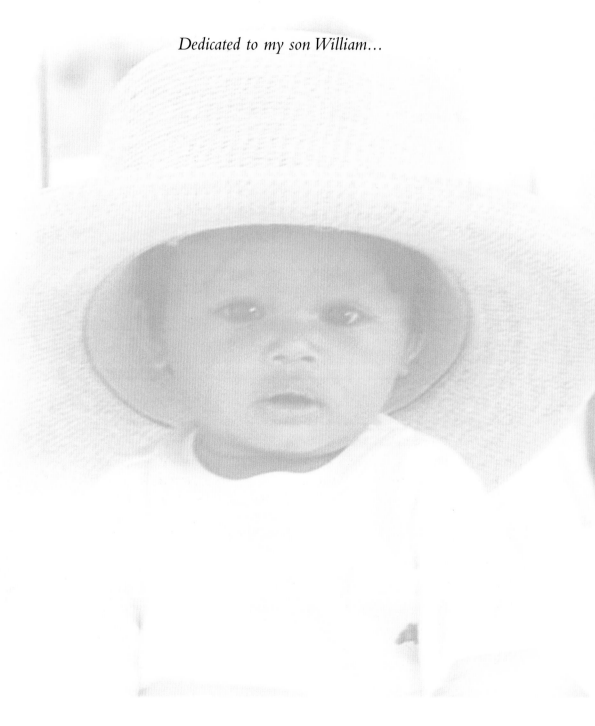

Foreword

When Dr. Bissoon asked me to write this forward, I was happy to accept. In this book, you will discover not just the causes, symptoms and treatments for cellulite, you will find valuable advice on everyday things you can do to prevent cellulite and increase the effectiveness of Mesotherapy. Dr. Bissoon offers simple, straightforward explanations of how this pioneering field of medicine can work for you.

I am truly blessed that Dr. Bissoon became part of my life. After just one year of treatment, I have witnessed a drastic reduction in my cellulite. My regimen of Mesotherapy, regular exercise and careful diet helped me shed more than 50 pounds, and has improved the appearance of my skin in those "troublesome areas" (with which most women are far too familiar). The whole process has given me tremendous joy, boosting my self-confidence and my self-image.

As an entertainer, I've always dealt with the usual fears, stresses and psychological constraints associated with being in the public eye. Couple this with my own hyper-criticism of my appearance, and you can imagine some of the burdens I've carried over the years. The success of Dr. Bissoon's treatment has made a direct and lasting impact on my life and career. It has allowed me to pursue my passions more fervently and confidently than before. Not only do I feel better overall, I feel better about myself!

Love and happiness!
Roberta Flack

Introduction
TO THE CELLULITE CURE

By Dr. Denise Bruner

Medical advances are born from those with an insatiable curiosity to explore new treatment models and methods. "The Cellulite Cure" reflects Dr. Lionel Bissoon's odyssey of discovery—one that resulted in an effective therapy to eradicate cellulite. Five years ago, Dr. Bissoon heeded the desperate pleas of a patient who insisted that he learn how to treat her cellulite with Mesotherapy. Although it was very popular in Europe and South America, Mesotherapy was virtually unknown in the United States. His sojourn took him to France to learn from the foremost Mesotherapy experts, including Dr. Michel Pistor, the discoverer of Mesotherapy. Since then, Dr. Bissoon has spearheaded the effort to establish Mesotherapy as a recognized medical specialty in the U.S.

As a bariatric physician (one who specializes in treating obesity and diseases associated with obesity), I have treated thousands of patients over the course of more than two decades. My dedication to finding innovative treatment strategies for my patients eventually led me to serve as the President of the American Society of Bariatric Physicians, a position I held for three years. Although I helped patients shed excess pounds, many were still embarrassed to wear short clothing because of unsightly cellulite. At first, my research on Mesotherapy yielded a paucity of information on its effectiveness as a cellulite treatment. Although I was skeptical, I refused to simply dismiss Mesotherapy as "snake oil."

My curiosity led me to a momentous meeting with Dr. Bissoon, one of the foremost practitioners and physician educators in the field. His revolutionary book, *The Cellulite Cure,* provides a detailed review of the history of cellulite, along with an easy to understand explanation of basic skin anatomy and physiology and the reasons for cellulite formation. Furthermore, he presents evidence- and results-based treatment. This cutting-edge information describes a new and unique solution that can be life transforming for the thousands who feel hopelessly disfigured by cellulite.

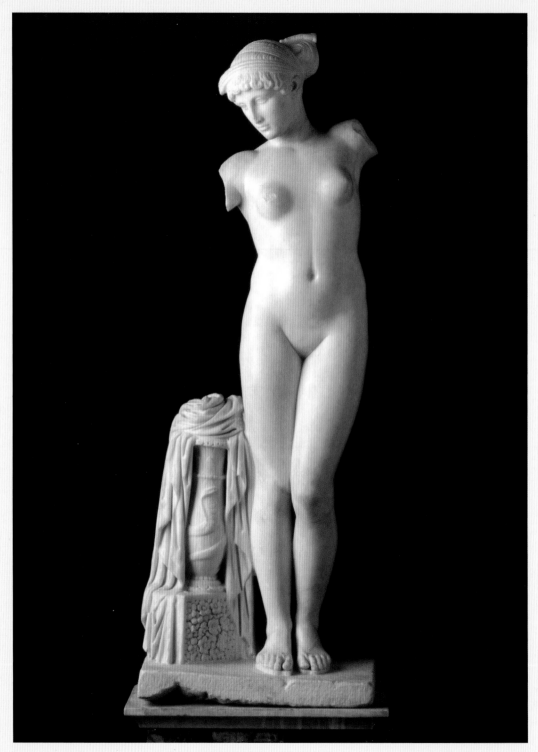

FIG. 1: "Esquiline Venus" 1ST Century Rome, Italy

1. *A Brief History of*
Cellulite

Unlike many maladies that have plagued human beings

for millennia, no anthropologist, historian or physician

knows when or where cellulite originated. Ancient

medical texts contain references to various illnesses,

treatments and parts of the anatomy, but no descrip-

tions of cellulite. The Greek physician Hippocrates says

nothing about dimpled thighs with the texture of

"orange peels." The historian Herodotus is mute on the

subject of buttocks that resemble "cottage cheese."

The ancient Egyptians, Greeks and Romans either chose

to depict women as smooth-skinned and blemish free,

or they did so because cellulite didn't exist. See Figure 1.

My observations of various lifestyles and cultures around the world suggest that cellulite is a fairly modern phenomenon. The medical condition is "modern" in the sense that women living in today's industrialized nations are more likely to exhibit symptoms than women in pre-industrial societies. Although 80%–90% of American women show signs of cellulite (to greater or lesser degrees), the condition is less common among women in hunter-gatherer societies. (I'll suggest explanations for this in Chapter 3.)

Whether the classical Greeks and Romans were "telling it like it was," or putting a positive spin on the female form, their ideal of feminine beauty was relatively thin, fit and free of cellulite. Because cellulite is barely mentioned in the medical literature of the 20TH century (or any other century), the only clues to its origin and evolution are in the paintings of artists such as Peter Paul Rubens (1577-1640) and photographers like Arthur Albert Allen (worked 1916-1930). In both cases, the documentation of cellulite was quite unintentional.

From the Baroque to the Bikini

Judging from the masterpieces of painters such as Rubens, plump women were fashionable during the Baroque period. So prized were Rubens' depictions of chubby female goddesses and nymphs that the term "Rubenesque" survives as a euphemism for attractive, overweight women. (Check any personal page or dating website if you don't believe me. See, for example, Figure 2.) In Rubens' paintings, we finally see evidence of cellulite. See Figures 3 and 5. Since then, other artists have depicted cellulite in tempera paints, oils, bronze and marble. Until fairly recently, female fat and cellulite were considered good things—a manifestation of a life dedicated to leisure. Artistic appreciation of plump female forms continued well into the 20TH century, and probably stemmed from several factors:

Attractive, rubenesque, intelligent woman with no dependents, seeks S/D/WPM 45-57 to share some morning walks/runs, afternoon lunches and evenings at theater, Lyric Opera, fine dining and home cooking/baking. You, like me, are a non-smoker, non-drug user (social drinker OK), cheery guy who is emotionally available and capable of warm, intimate relationships, and spiritually and financially healthy. You are also a successful, degreed, professional

Fig. 2

The women who served as models were often well fed.

Excess pounds meant you were wealthy and living the "good life."

Peasant women and factory workers were often less attractive because they had no time to visit beauty salons and spas.

With the invention of photography in 1839, artists had a new medium to capture their visions, and it didn't take long (one year) before the first nude was photographed. Although early photographic nudes display portly women, my evaluations revealed no evidence of cellulite on the subjects' thighs and buttocks. Is this because early equipment and lighting was not sophisticated enough to capture cellulite on film? I doubt it. The photos were taken from different angles, which could have easily revealed any cellulite. Therefore, I'm willing to believe these women had no cellulite. Unlike Rubens' subjects, however, these models appear to be members of the working class.

American photographer Arthur Albert Allen, took over four thousand nude photographs that detail the skin's appearance on models ranging from portly to slim. Upon close examination, there is little evidence of cellulite. See Figure 4. When it appears, it's limited to the saddlebag areas and buttocks, where the condition first manifests. (As the disease progresses, it appears around the knees.) Allen's work has proven invaluable to the study of cellulite, though it was not universally appreciated. On several occasions, officials who could not distinguish

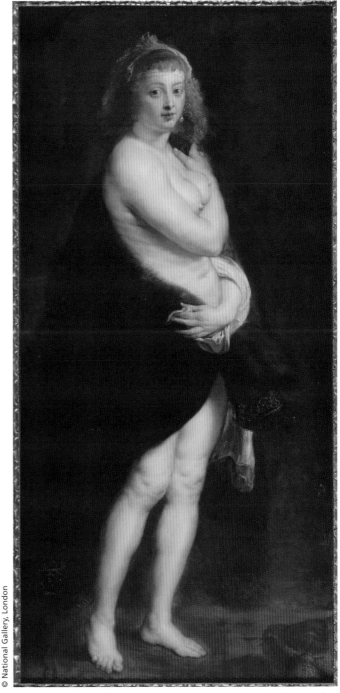

Fɪɢ. 3: One of the masterpieces by Peter Paul Rubens: "The Little Fur"

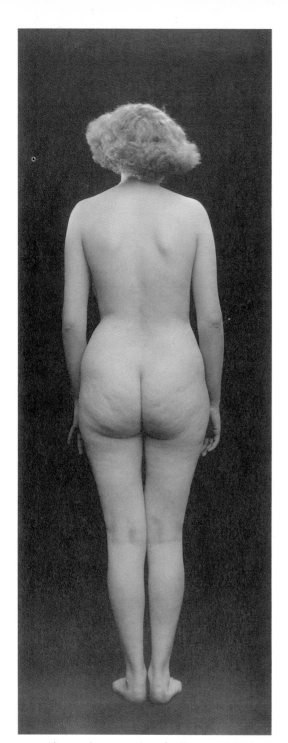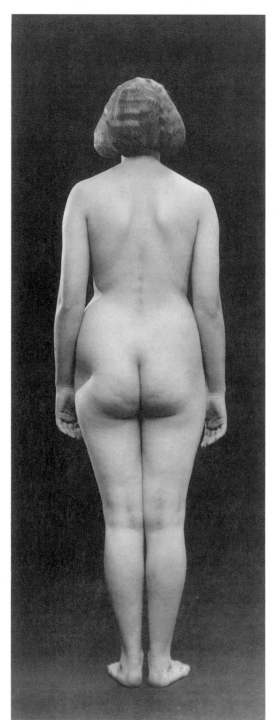

FIG. 4: These photographs of Allen models show evidence of cellulite.

between nudity and pornography jailed him.

To record and illustrate my points about cellulite, I will also employ a series of photographs.

Although the preference for portly women reigned for hundreds of years (see also Figure 6), "thin was in" by the latter half of the 20TH century. As hemlines became shorter, and swimwear grew more scandalous, society revised its notions of feminine beauty. Lithe and athletic was the new paradigm. You'll still find people who go "zowie for zaftig," but most Westerners strive for a body that is thin, unwrinkled and cellulite free.

It was only when women became braver, and began to wear revealing clothes that cellulite became an issue.

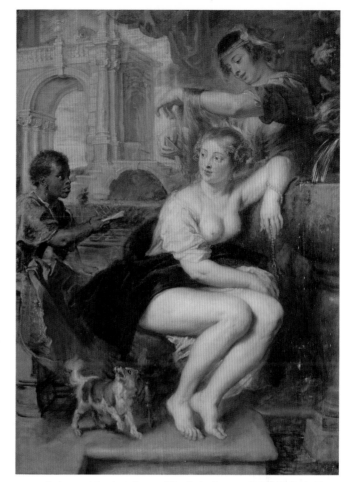

FIG. 5: Rubens Masterpiece: "Bathsheba at the Fountain"
© Staatliche Kunstsammlungen, Dresden

By reviewing over 150 years of photographs, we see a slow evolution of the swimsuit and its hemlines. The next photo (Figure 7) shows a Chicago police officer measuring a woman's swimsuit to determine if she has violated any local and state laws. Although the bikini was first unveiled in Paris in 1946, (Figure 8) it was not until the late '60s and '70s that it became common beachwear.

By the 1960s, bikinis, short shorts and miniskirts exposed female thighs for all to see—probably for the first time since gladiators hacked away in the Roman Coliseum. Suddenly, dimpled thighs and buttocks with a "mattress" texture didn't

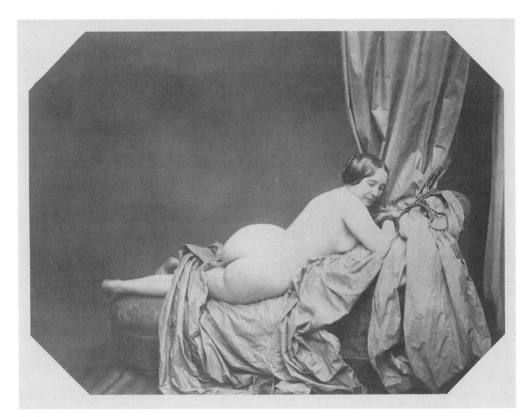

Fɪɢ. 6

© Cleveland Museum of Art

represent the high life, but were a cause for embarrassment, anxiety and mental anguish.

It was only when women became braver, and began to wear revealing clothes that cellulite became an issue. It brought much more awareness to the condition than ever before. We went from a culture that didn't have much body exposure to a culture that walked around in G-strings and thongs on the beach. For this reason, I sometimes think of cellulite as a new disease. Last century's beauty rage is this century's plague.

Cellulite first gained widespread attention in 1973, thanks largely to Nicole Ronsard's best-selling book, *Cellulite: Those Lumps, Bumps and Bulges You Couldn't Lose Before*. By this time, women had become more courageous in terms of fashion: the bikini was now common beach attire, and miniskirts and hot pants ruled the streets. Ironically, just as women began revealing more skin, diets were changing for the worse. The 1970s witnessed the birth of

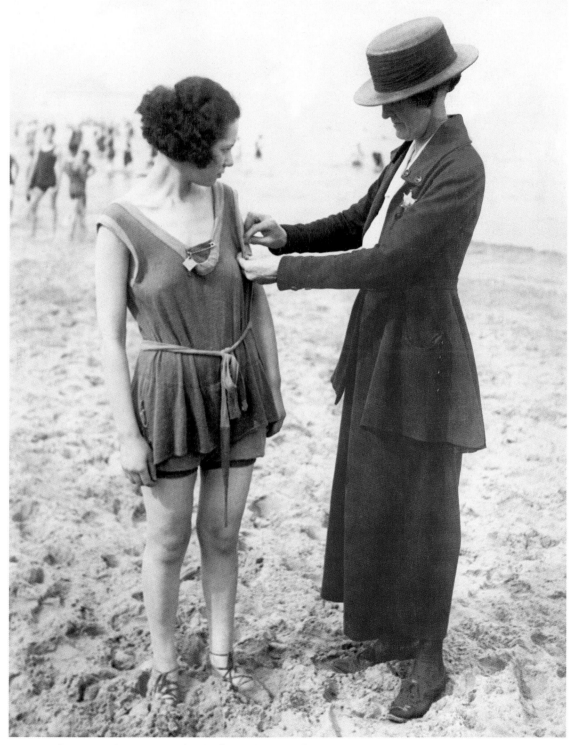

Fɪɢ. 7: A Chicago policewoman checks for violations of the bathing suit length laws in 1921.

© Corbis Images

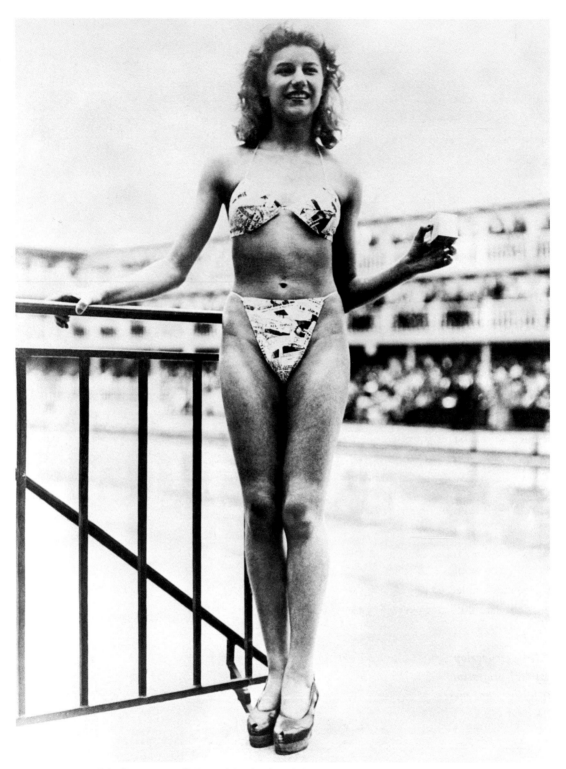

FIG. 8: Dancer Micheline Bernardini models the first bikini at a contest, July 11, 1946 in Paris, France.

© Corbis Images

the Standard American Diet (S.A.D.)—a diet skewed toward processed foods laden with fat, sugar and preservatives. In addition, many people adopted more sedentary lifestyles during the last 25 years, thanks to the proliferation of PCs, cable TV and video games. Both trends have conspired to transform Americans into the fattest people on Earth.

Is it any wonder that 90% of the female population is now preoccupied with cellulite—how to hide it, reduce it or eliminate it?

Patent Medicine

Some of my patients believe that if 80 to 90% of men developed cellulite, medical science would have invented a cure by the time Rubens painted the dimpled hips on his nymphs.

I disagree. If men were predisposed to cellulite, they *might* have looted countless treasuries *trying* to discover a cure, but they would have failed. They would have failed for the same reasons they failed to invent cures for baldness and impotence until the late 20TH century. The science and technology simply weren't there.

(Men <u>can</u> develop cellulite, but the condition is quite rare. Some medical professionals classify male "cellulite" as a separate condition that merely <u>resembles</u> female cellulite. See Figure 9.)

In fact, various "treatments" for cellulite have been marketed for decades. Different creams, lotions, aromatherapy, exercise and

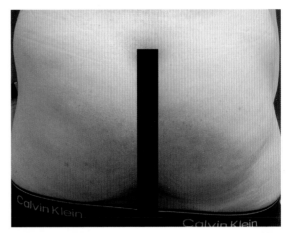
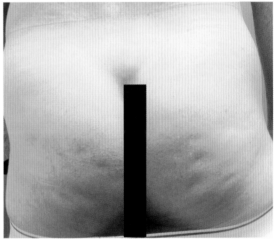

FIG. 9: The man shown here with cellulite was treated with Subcision™. Note his *before (bottom)* and *after (top)*.

Lionel Bissoon

massage therapies have all been touted as potential "solutions." Conduct an Internet search using the keyword "cellulite," and you'll get thousands of hits for articles, essays and ads touting these cellulite "solutions." What you won't find is a product or process that actually works. Creams, lotions, manual massage and mechanical massage devices are not genuine cures, because they only reduce the *appearance* of cellulite; they don't *cure* the condition by addressing the underlying causes. And the causes of cellulite *are* underlying—they literally take place beneath the surface of the skin, below the epidermis.

The popularity of cellulite creams mushroomed after Frank Greenway, M.D. and his colleagues published a landmark article entitled "Topical Fat Reduction" in 1995, which helped spawn an entire industry. The authors studied the effects of aminophylline, forskolin and yohimbine as topical fat-reduction ointments—individually and in combination. The results, which proved that aminophyilline was most effective in breaking down fat, boosted widespread use of the aminophylline thigh cream for cellulite.

The only creams and lotions that provide some relief are those containing liposomes, which allow medications to penetrate the skin. However, most products with liposomes target only the fat cells. Reducing the size of fat cells and ignoring the other two aspects of cellulite formation produces only temporary relief. Therefore, I recommend a product called Mesolysis™, which treats all three cellulite "culprits."

Cellulite forms when fat cells protrude abnormally ("herniate") through the connective tissue of the fat lobes (See Chapter 2). Some factors that cause cellulite include weakened microcirculation of the blood, poor lymphatic drainage and damaged connective tissues in the affected areas. Poor circulation and retention of lymphatic fluids allows toxins to accumulate in

Creams, lotions and mechanical massages are not genuine cellulite cures. They reduce the appearance of cellulite without addressing the underlying causes.

various fat and skin cells, initiating a "domino effect of damage" that eventually results in cellulite. Although medicine does not yet fully understand how the various factors work together to produce cellulite, it is known that the hormone estrogen—in combination with certain diets, clothing and lack of exercise—contributes to the problem. *(I'll discuss the causes and development of cellulite in Chapter 2.)*

Mesotherapy: The Cellulite Cure™

Understandably, most women are embarrassed when their hips, thighs and buttocks resemble cottage cheese, orange peels or mattresses. Even the terms used to describe the condition are insulting. How many of you feel comfortable wearing bikinis when cellulite mars your appearance? Isn't cellulite something that only fat women get—or senior citizens? If your thighs look like the surface of the moon, you must be doing something wrong. Right?

Wrong.

Isn't cellulite something that only fat women get—or senior citizens? If your thighs look like the surface of the moon, you must be doing something wrong.

Nearly all women, regardless of their age, weight, height or ethnic background can fall victim to cellulite. Although cellulite does involve the herniation of fat cells, obesity has nothing to do with "cottage cheese" production. In fact, cellulite tends to be more pronounced in "skinny" women, while some obese women "wear it" pretty well.

Although most women are genetically predisposed to cellulite, it's important to note that "predisposition" is not the same as "destiny." The appearance of this medical condition is not

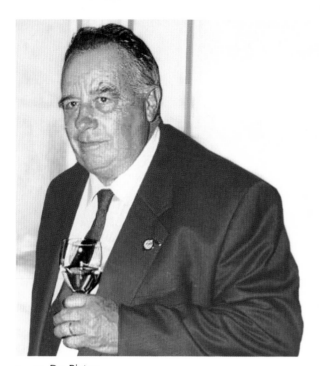

Fig. 10: Dr. Pistor

Photo courtesy of Dr. Petit, France

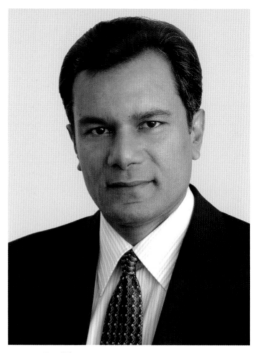

Fig. 11: Dr. Bissoon

© Steven Ladner

inevitable. And if it does occur, you no longer have to live with it, thanks to a medical treatment known as Mesotherapy. Mesotherapy treats the cottage cheese appearance of skin. Mesotherapy Stringcision™ is designed for dimples, and Surgical Subcision™ eliminates rimples. ("Meso" literally means "middle," and refers to the mesoderm, where the treatment is administered). ***Rimples are the fine, shallow linear horizontal elongated depressions in the back of the thighs.*** (See sample in Figure 12.)

The medical specialty of Mesotherapy was discovered by French physician Dr. Michel Pistor (see Figure 10) during the 1950s, and has long been been employed in France and elsewhere to treat a variety of ailments—most notably for the pain and trauma caused by sports-related injuries. In the half century since this medical specialty was first pioneered by Dr. Pistor, physicians such as Dr. Christian Chams, Dr. Elizabeth Dancey, Dr. Maurice Drae (and myself in the U.S.A.) have pioneered cosmetic Mesotherapy techniques to spur weight loss, treat hair loss and aging skin, and (of course) eliminate cellulite.

As part of his Topical Fat Reduction study, Dr. Greenway also injected isoproterenol into the thighs of patients, which demonstrated the medication's effectiveness in producing changes in leg girth. Unknowingly, the researchers were performing Mesotherapy. Today, their article is acknowledged as the first English-language publication on Mesotherapy, and it still forms the basis for almost all Mesotherapy formulas used in America to treat weight loss and cellulite. Therefore, Greenway and his colleagues can rightfully claim to be the "Founding Fathers of American Mesotherapy."

Mesotherapy involves multiple hypodermic injections of small doses of pharmaceuticals, homeopathic medications and vitamins into the mesoderm, or middle dermis, the tissue layer located just beneath the skin. This tissue layer contains stem cells, a type of rejuvenating cell that can transform into new healthy connective tissue, as well as adipocytes or fat cells. Mesotherapy is a multi-faceted approach to successfully treating cellulite—one that offers significant advantages over methods such as liposuction.

A study that appeared in a 2000 issue of *Plastic and Reconstructive Surgery* reported a death rate of about 20 in every 100,000 patients who underwent liposuction between 1994 and 1998. This number is higher than the United States' death rate for motor vehicle accidents during that period! Liposuction has undergone some improvement since the "bad old days"— the 1970s—when death rates were eight times higher.

It's important to note that no reported deaths have occurred as a result of Mesotherapy, despite decades of use with hundreds of thousands of patients. What's more, very few infections have occurred, and most (if not all) were probably caused by unskilled Mesotherapists.

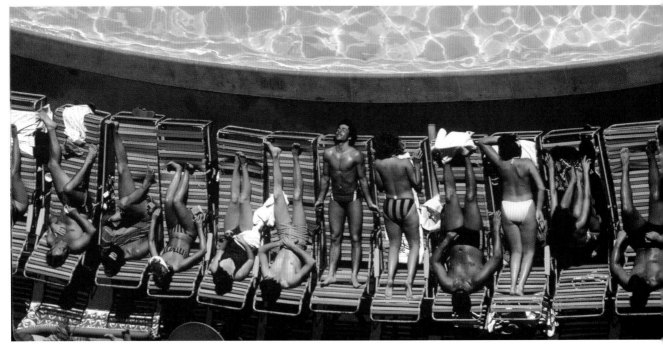

Fig. 12: Sample of *rimples* can be seen from above.
© Stephen Trimble

The skilled Mesotherapist easily and safely delivers a tailor-made mixture of medications that elicits numerous beneficial responses in the mesoderm and underlying fatty tissue. One benefit is an increase in blood flow to the tissues, which brings vital oxygen and nutrients to the fibroblasts that secrete and maintain connective tissue. Healthy connective tissue literally "connects" the underlying fat cells into properly arranged bundles or lobules. A lobule of fat cells that is intact and structurally sound generates a smooth and appealing topography on the outer dermis—smooth external skin.

Another benefit: when the proper mixture of lipolytics (lipo = fat; lytic = dissolve) permeates the mesoderm, it can literally dissolve underlying fat cells, "melting" away cells that primarily give rise to cellulite. Still another benefit is a softening of connective tissues, a reversal of the hardening (sclerosis) that often accompanies age and waning hormone levels. Finally,

Mesotherapy improves lymphatic drainage from the cellulitic tissues. Lymph is the fluid that normally drains from all bodily tissues, returning to large vessels that eventually make their way to the heart for recirculation and re-oxygenation.

Mesotherapy is a direct and highly effective approach to treating the disease, not just a temporary remission of the symptoms. Mesotherapy is a *real* cure, not a palliative treatment that only assuages the mind of the patient. Mesotherapy cannot be purchased over the counter in bottles or boxes or even by prescription. There are no at-home Mesotherapy kits available for a few dollars. The current treatment is a modern, high-tech, biologic modifier approach that involves multiple visits to the doctor's office, and takes weeks or months to complete. The good news is that Mesotherapy produces *amazing* results in reducing and/or eliminating cellulite. The average patient will require 10-15 treatment sessions with a once per year follow-up.

It *really* works—in the hands of a skilled physician who is experienced in the techniques and biological modifiers.

I have personally treated hundreds of patients, and witnessed one success story after another using Mesotherapeutic techniques and medicines. *(See the story of Pamela, following.)*

Pills, lotions, hand massages, mechanical massages and applications of various creams or the use of certain exercise machines may claim this kind of success, but they do not deliver on their promises. The successes you'll read about in the numerous patient testimonials and conclusive before/after photos in this book are extraordinarily convincing.

I will show you how Mesotherapy—in combination with simple, easy-to-follow changes in your habits and lifestyle—can elimi-nate, or at least dramatically reduce, the extent and degree of your cellulite. I'll provide a detailed explanation of what causes cellulite and how the "domino effect of damage" can progress if left untreated. Most important, I'll explain how Mesotherapy works, and why the availability of this technique/medical specialty means that thousands of women like you no longer have to live with the embarrassment and mental stress of cellulite. Living with cellulite is now a matter of choice—not an inevitable consequence of being a woman.

In the subsequent chapters, I'll also explain how to facilitate the Cellulite Cure by combining the Mesotherapy procedures known as Subcision™ and Mesotherapy Stringcision™. These procedures can reduce the number of treatment sessions by 65% to 75%, and yield more "instant gratification." They provide accelerated cures for many women when the condition involved is limited to dimpling and rimples. ⬦

Living with cellulite is now a matter of choice—not an inevitable consequence of being a woman.

A Letter from "Pamela"

"I always remember having it—even during my teenage years," says Pamela of her cellulite. "It was on my thighs: the insides. My mother and sister also have it. We call it 'the curse.'"

Now 55, Pamela lives on Long Island, and remains actively involved in sports and exercise, including biking, horseback riding and windsurfing. Unfortunately, her cellulite continued to worsen as she grew older, and became more severe during pregnancy, her menstrual cycles and at menopause.

"I never wore shorts or skirts above the knee. And it shows through white clothes, so that was something to think about. If I didn't have it, I would have been an athlete, a swimmer, but I didn't want anyone to see me in a suit." Interestingly, Pamela found that men seemed to care less about her cellulite than women. "My husband couldn't care less, but women noticed: there were snickers and little remarks."

"I tried medicines and creams, and it helped, but not like [Mesotherapy]. I also tried special massage…and endermologie a few times."

"After reading about Mesotherapy in a magazine, and asking about the procedure at a local spa, I decided to give it a try. Initially, I wanted to have my back and abdomen treated. I had grown accustomed to living with the cellulite so I opted not to treat my legs. I was so thrilled with the results of my new waist that I decided to try the Mesotherapy for my cellulite. The doctor claimed he could improve my legs. Well, he was right. The results were immediate and within three sessions my legs were perfect!"

"Mesotherapy [can be] painful and scary-looking, but I would definitely recommend it. This gives you hope!"

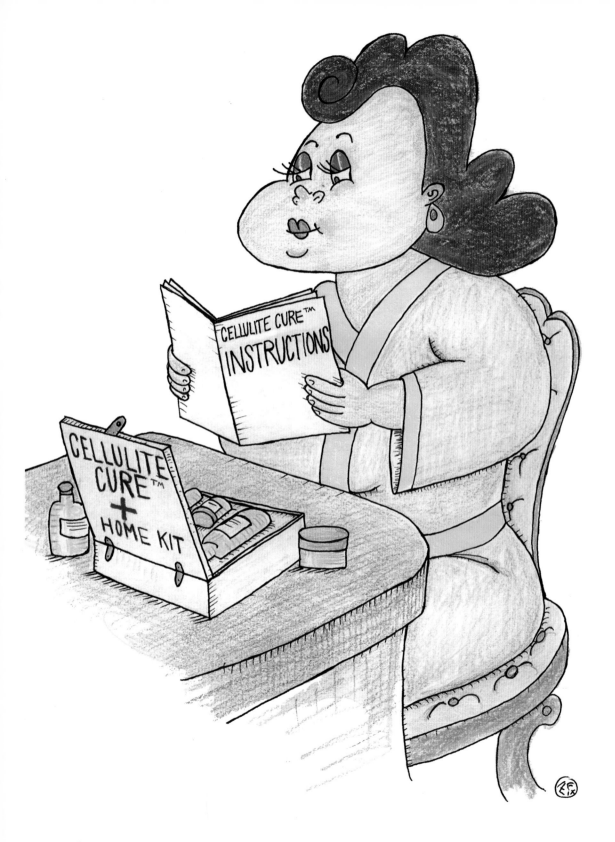

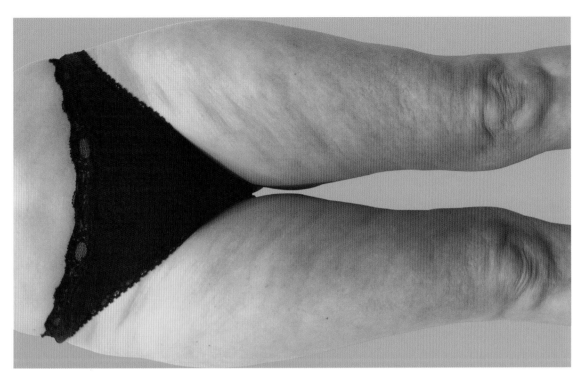

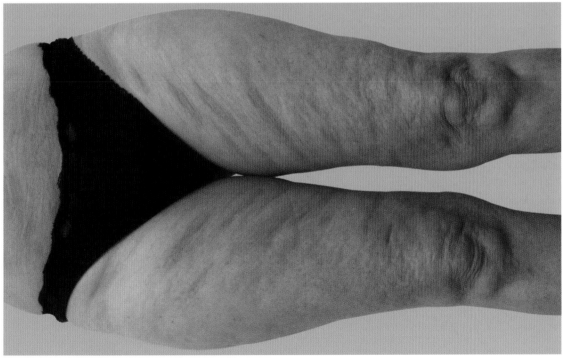

FIG. 13A-13B: This woman was treated with three sessions of Mesotherapy in conjunction with the Mesolysis™ Cellulite cream. (*Bottom/left* shows her *before*, *top/right* photo shows *after*.)

Lionel Bissoon

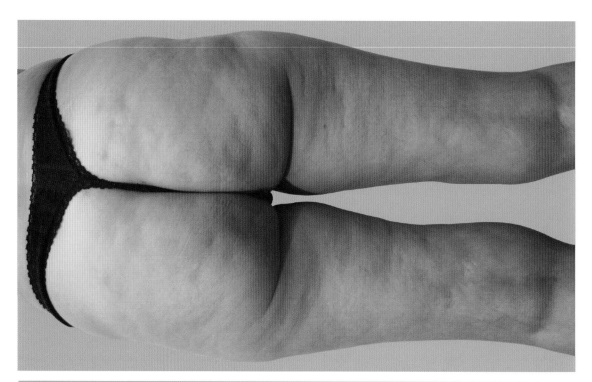

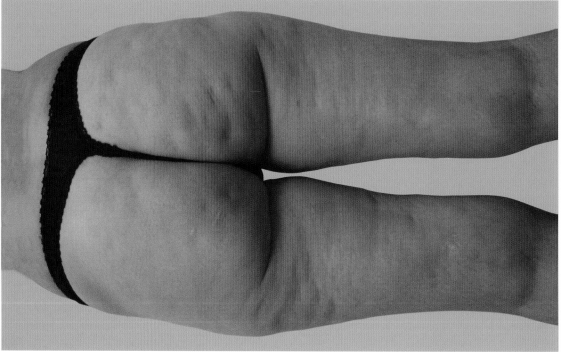

FIG. **14A-14B**: This is the same patient, her *back* view. The bottom photo is *before*, top *after.*

Lionel Bissoon

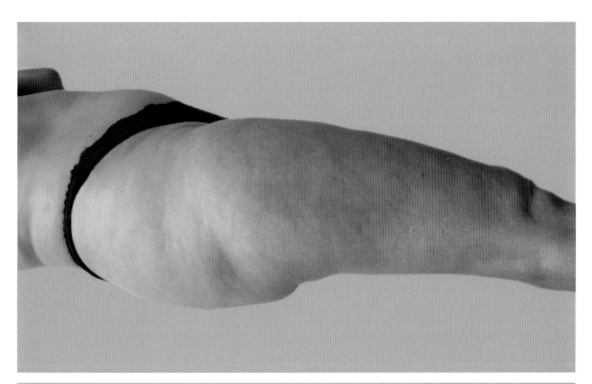

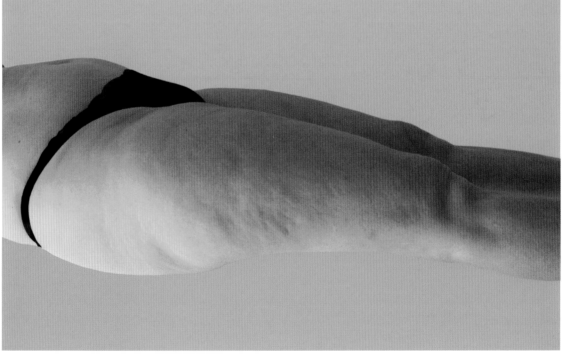

FIG. 15A-15B: This is the same patient. Bottom photo is *before*, the top is *after*.
Lionel Bissoon

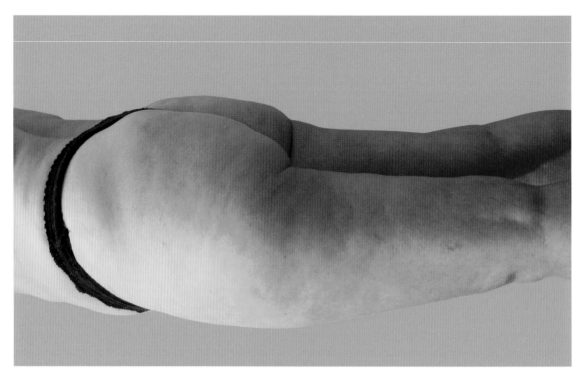

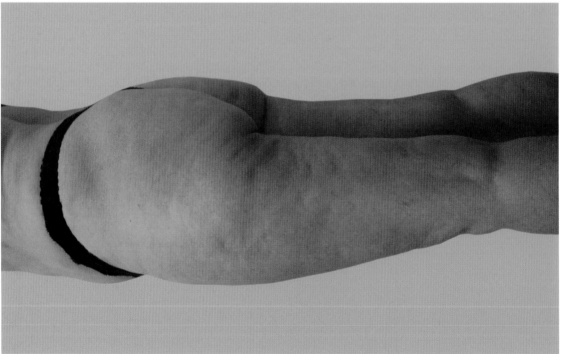

FIG. 16A-16B: These photos show the same patient. The bottom photo is *before*, the top is *after*.

Lionel Bissoon

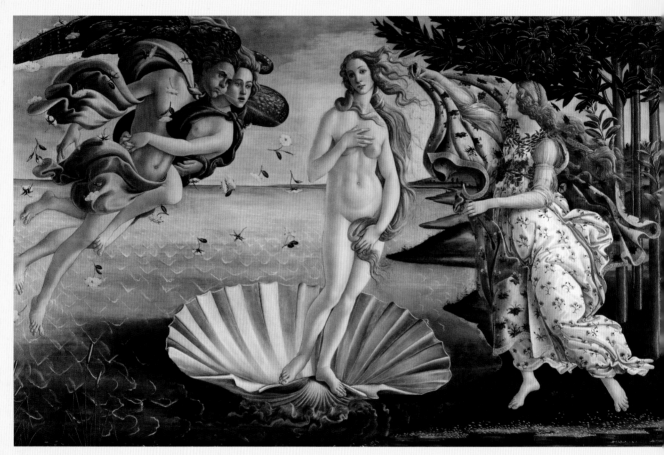

Fig. 1: "Birth of Venus" by Sandro Botticelli circa 1478-1487

© Corbis Images

2. *Skin Anatomy* 101

Before discussing the hows and whys of cellulite

formation, it's important to have a basic understanding

of your skin's anatomy and physiology. Once you know

the basics of skin structure—how healthy skin should

look, feel and function—it's easier to comprehend

how changes to the structure and physiology can lead

to cellulite. If it seems that my lecture in "Skin Anatomy

101" touches on topics that have little to do with

cellulite, please bear with me. The process of cellulite

formation will become *crystal clear* once I've supplied

a little background.

Although many authors have studied the microscopic and visible anatomy of cellulite, F. Mirrashed and his colleagues, Michael Rosenbaum, M.D. and his team offer the best modern descriptions. Mirrashed used MRI imaging to describe the anatomy, while Rosenbaum analyzed tissue samples from cellulite patients. For the sake of brevity, I'll limit my discussion to the key factors that cause cellulite development in women.

The skin is the largest organ in the human body.

The skin is the largest organ in the human body. Like most paper towels, your skin has a "two-ply" structure composed of the outer layer, the epidermis, and a thicker, lower layer called the dermis. In addition to skin cells, the dermis contains nerves, blood vessels, lymphatic vessels, glands and hair follicles. See Figure 2.

Taken together, the components of the epidermis and dermis work to protect you from the external environment by: preventing water absorption and water loss; absorbing and blocking radiation; regulating your internal temperature, and giving you the sense of touch.

The components of the epidermis and dermis work to protect you from the external environment.

As you probably know, the epidermis is extremely thin (ranging from .02 to .04 millimeters, or an average of $1/1000^{TH}$ of an inch), and continuously renews itself by shedding surface cells in a process called "desquamation" or "exfoliation." Although exfoliation slows down after age 30, human beings shed their entire skin numerous times during their lives.

Prior to age 30, the skin is shed every 30 days, but shedding becomes less frequent after this, occurring every 45-50 days. On numerous occasions, I've seen new patients who complain of cellulite when their true affliction was actually a "crepe-like" skin

Prior to age 30, the skin is shed every 30 days, but shedding becomes less frequent after this— 45-50 days.

Epidermis —

Dermis —

Hypodermis —
(Superficial
Fascia)

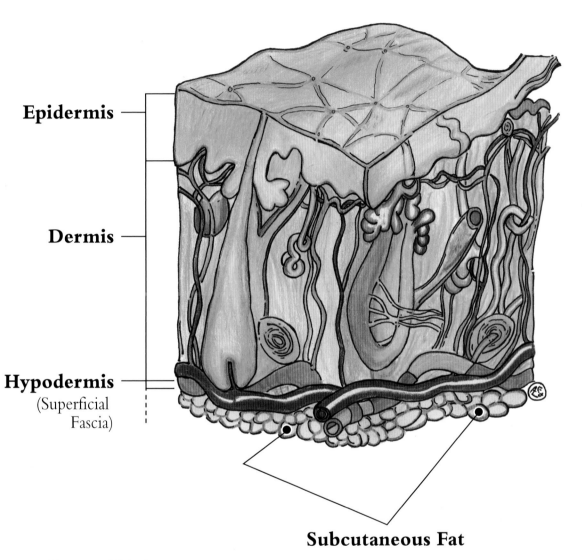

Subcutaneous Fat

<small>Fig. 2:</small> Diagram of Skin Anatomy

texture on the thighs. Crepe-like skin is not cellulite. It's caused by layers of dead skin that have accumulated instead of being shed. To promote "turnover" of healthy skin layer, I suggest a 10% glycolic cream or 10% glycolic pad formulation which facilitates regular exfoliation and removal of fine lines.

Coating your skin with acid may sound drastic, but fear not. Glycolic acid is nothing more than a fruit acid commonly referred to as an alpha hydroxy. In this formulation, the natural acid—when applied according to the directions— is safe and effective. It loosens the gluey substances that hold the outer layer of dead (often damaged) skin to the inner layers of younger, smoother skin waiting to migrate outward. To promote turnover of the healthy skin layer, I suggest a 10% glycolic cream formulation which facilitates regular exfoliation and removal of fine lines. The glycolic acid peel/cream may produce a burning sensation in some patients which also increases collagen production and skin toning.

Blood & Lymph Circulation

The base of the epidermis serves as both a boundary layer and an interface with the dermis, which itself is a multi-layered structure composed of connective tissue that is about two millimeters thick. Within the dermis, tiny blood vessels (capillaries) supply oxygen and nutrients to many cells. To appreciate the difference between veins, capillaries and lymphatic vessels, think of veins as your blood's interstate highways, with capillaries serving as one-lane roads, and lymphatic vessels as dirt paths and hiking trails.

Unlike the arteries—your bloodstream's "superhighways"—veins, capillaries and lymphatic vessels contain *smooth* muscles within their walls to return blood to general circulation after it's traveled to every cell in the body. Instead, smaller circulatory "highways" rely on three factors to return blood—now deoxygenated and containing carbon dioxide and other toxic materials—to the heart and lungs. These are: the plantar return reflex, which pumps blood from the legs back into the pelvis; the thoraco-abdominal pump; and the muscles.

The Plantar Return Reflex. This is a reflex area located in the sole of the foot that stimulates the return of lymph. People often trigger this reflex unconsciously by stamping their feet when they've been standing still for long periods of time—cashiers, security guards, cops on the beat, etc. See Figure 3 and Figure 4 following.

The Thoraco-Abdominal Pump.
The diaphragm is a small muscle that separates the chest from the abdomen. When you breathe, the diaphragm travels downward, creating negative pressure in the chest cavity (a vacuum) that helps pull deoxygenated blood and lymphatic fluids into the heart. The diaphragm also produces positive pressure in the abdomen (squeezing), which also forces blood back into the chest. In other words, the diaphragm has two functions: it creates negative pressure in the chest and positive pressure in the abdomen. Both functions work in concert to return blood and lymph to the heart. See Figure 4.

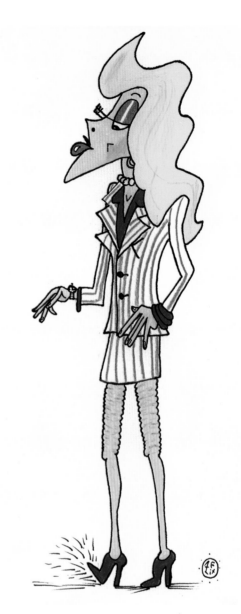

Fɪɢ. 3: Activation of the Plantar Reflex by Tapping of the Feet

Muscles. Muscles, which exert pressure on the veins and lymph vessels when contracted, surround the blood vessels in your legs, forcing blood and lymph back to the heart. On the outbound trip, fluid within the blood passes through the walls of the

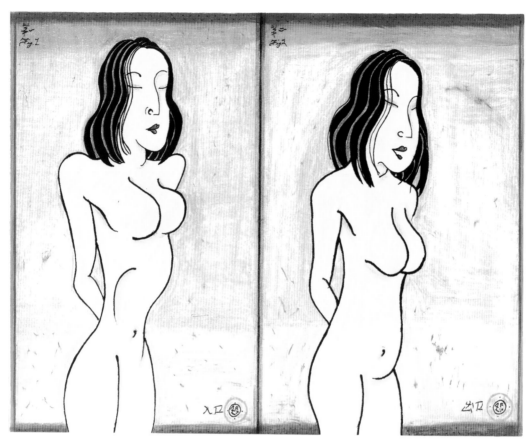

FIG. 4: When your diaphragm contracts in breathing, it descends and creates negative pressure in the thorax (chest), which creates a sucking action.

capillaries, and seeps into the tissues, providing them with nutrients and oxygen. On the return trip, veins return deoxygenated blood while lymph vessels remove the tissue fluids. The lymph vessels join to form larger vessels until they finally return lymph to general circulation from a connecting network in the groin for the lower body. In the groin, the lymph fluids are filtered by lymph nodes prior to entering the torso.

Connective Tissue. Connective tissue is the skeleton, the supporting structure for the dermis. It can be compared to a viscous gel whose consistency varies according to factors such as age, genetics, temperature and even mechanical stimulation (such as massage). One group of cells that compose connective tissue is commonly called fibroblasts, and two of their functions are to produce collagen and elastin.

Collagen makes up 70% of the dermis, and gives the skin structural support for the cells and blood vessels. Collagen also allows the skin to stretch and contract, which aids in the healing of wounds. Elastin occupies the spaces between collagen fibers, and provides elasticity and resiliency to the skin. Elastin degrades slowly, but steadily, and must be replaced by new elastin.

The dermis also contains large molecules called glycosamino-glycans and proteoglycans (you don't have to pronounce those) that retain and release water, and are responsible for regulating the skin's turgor—in other words, its normal rigidity and surface tension.

Damage to connective tissue makes it weaker and less elastic, and is a major factor in cellulite formation.

When fibroblasts are starved of oxygen and vital nutrients, and veins and lymph vessels are unable to drain the tissues effectively, fluid builds up between cells and protein within the fluid settles out to form thick and inelastic fibers between fat cells. As they become unhealthy, the fibroblasts fail to remove abnormal protein fibers, and to rebuild collagen and elastin fibers. Pressure builds up within the tissue, causing it to feel hard, tender and lumpy. Blood cannot pass through the rigid, dense tissue freely. Instead the flow is decreased, causing the situation to worsen.

Put simply, once cellulite formation begins, it snowballs into a self-perpetuating cycle that is impossible to stop using conventional treatments.

Collagen makes up 70% of the dermis, and gives the skin structural support for the cells and blood vessels.

Fat

Earlier in this chapter, I referred to a boundary between the epidermis and dermis. In reality, there is no definite separation between the two skin layers. Instead, elements of the epidermis gradually blend into the dermis. Along with the dermis' connective tissue, there are fat cells called "adipocytes." These fat cells comprise a layer generally referred to as the subcutaneous fat layer, which covers the entire body, except for the eyelids.

The fat cells in the subcutaneous fat layer are organized into chambers (fat lobes), and are surrounded by connective tissue in a vertical fashion. The connective tissues bordering these fat chambers are called "septa." As I mentioned in Chapter 1, most women are predisposed to cellulite, whereas the condition is quite rare in men. See Figure 6A and B.

One reason is this: the structure of the dermis is different in women than in men. See Figure 8.

In a nutshell, women have larger fat lobes, and these fat lobes and septa have a different pattern in women than in men. In addition, women are much more efficient at storing energy in the form of fat and at releasing "fat energy" when needed (this is discussed in detail later). This difference gives women the ability to store fat during pregnancy. It also means that it's easier to gain weight and harder to shed excess pounds. See Figures 6A and B and Figure 7A and B.

More Fat

The subcutaneous fat layer is responsible for the appearance of cellulite in women. Worse: the fat layer is mainly regulated by hormones, and does not readily respond to diet and exercise. Liposuction cannot be performed at this level to reduce fat or

Once cellulite formation begins, it snowballs into a self-perpetuating cycle that is impossible to stop using conventional treatments.

HEALTHY SUPERFICIAL FAT LAYER AND SUBCUTANEOUS TISSUE

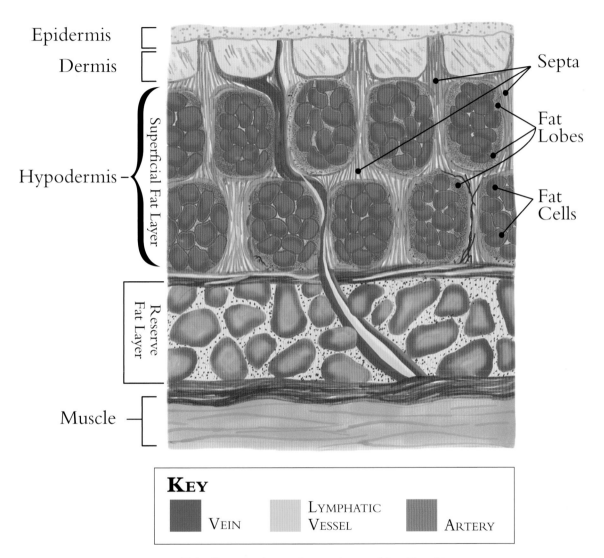

FIG. 5: This diagram shows the anatomy of healthy skin—the normal structure of fat/skin/circulation/dermis.

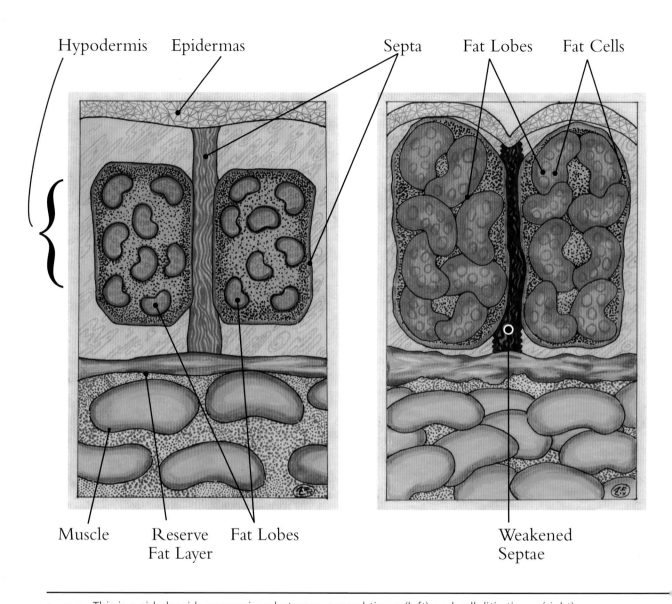

Hypodermis   Epidermas   Septa   Fat Lobes   Fat Cells

Muscle   Reserve   Fat Lobes   Weakened
              Fat Layer   Septae

FIG. 6A-6B: This is a side by side comparison between normal tissue (left) and cellulitic tissue (right).

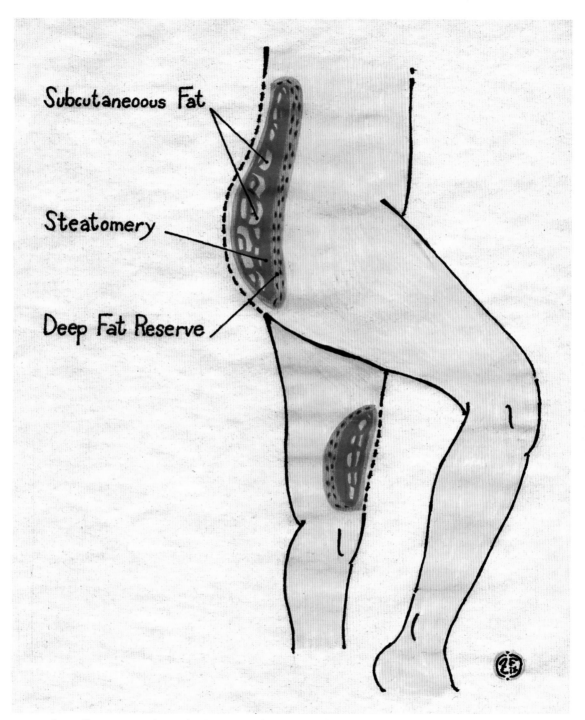

Subcutaneoous Fat

Steatomery

Deep Fat Reserve

FIG. 7A: These illustrations show the location of the three fat layers present in women.

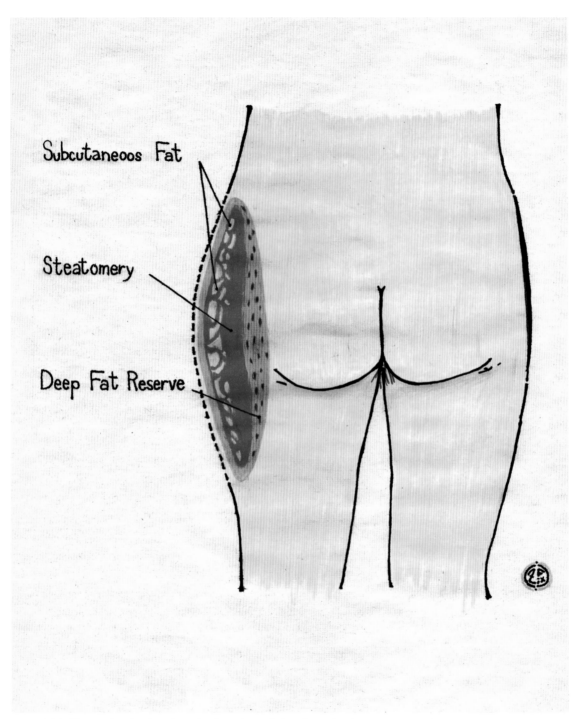

Subcutaneoos Fat

Steatomery

Deep Fat Reserve

FIG. 7B: This illustration is showing the location of the three fat layers present in women.

cellulite. When liposuction is performed in this area, it actually makes the appearance of the cellulite worse. This is why many women complain that liposuction exacerbates their cellulite. As if that weren't bad enough, women (unlike men) have an additional fat layer located underneath the subcutaneous fat layer. Known as the Superficial Reserve Fat Layer, or "Alimentary Fat Layer," the fat cells in this layer are *not* organized into defined fat chambers, and will respond to diet and exercise. This layer is the main target for liposuction.

Wait… I'm not finished with fat. There is yet another fat layer present only in women called the Deep Reserve Fat Layer, or "Steatomery." This layer occurs in specific areas of the female

Female	Male
Three fat layers are in buttocks, abdomen and knees.	One fat layer is throughout the body.
Thinner Skin	Thicker Skin
No cross-linking of underlying connective tissue (weaker)	Cross linked underlying connective tissue (stronger)
Ratio of beta receptors (break-down fat) to alpha receptors (fat storage) is 1:7 from the waist down.	The ratio of beta receptors to alpha receptors is 1:1.
Estrogen stimulates fat storage.	Testosterone breaks down fat.
Female fat cells are larger.	Male fat cells are smaller.

FIG. 8: A Comparison between Male and Female Fat and Connective Tissue

body—notably the *hips, lower abdomen, inner knees* and *the triceps brachial area.* Medical science commonly refers to this layer as the fat depot. Like the subcutaneous fat layer, this fat layer does not respond to diet and exercise. It does respond to starvation after a minimum of six months (great news, right?) and can also be reduced with liposuction.

Research by P. Mauriege and colleagues have demonstrated that there are seven alpha receptors (fat storing) for every beta receptor (betas break fat down). Thus, fat cells in the buttocks, thighs and knees have a greater proportion of fat-storing alpha-2 receptors, and a smaller percentage of fat-releasing beta receptors, than fat cells located elsewhere in the body. Fat cells in the cellulite-prone areas are not just hungrier for fat, they're far less likely to burn that fat in response to dieting and exercise. In fact, the ability of cells in the thighs and buttocks to release fat is just one-sixth that of all other fat cells. See Figures 9A and B.

In other words, for every seven pounds you gain, six will gravitate to your thighs and buttocks; just one pound will find another home. For every seven pounds you lose, only one will be shed from the problem areas, while six will melt from other regions.

What about Cellulite?

What does all of this have to do with cellulite? Here's where the background information pays off.

1. If you've ever wondered why women tend to acquire excess fat on their thighs, hips and abdomen, now you know. Women have more fat layers than men, and these layers are resistant to diet and exercise. In addition, fat layers such as the subcutaneous one cannot be treated with liposuction.

2. Poor blood circulation and lymphatic drainage can lead to fluid retention and damage connective tissues in the subcutaneous fat layer, causing them to become "sclerotic" (hardened). In turn, this negatively impacts the ability

The fat layer is mainly regulated by hormones, and does not readily respond to diet and exercise.

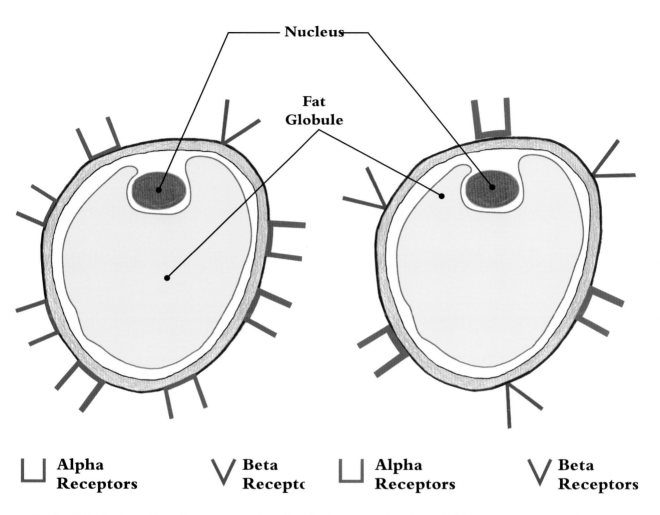

Nucleus

Fat Globule

Alpha Receptors   Beta Receptc   Alpha Receptors   Beta Receptors

G. 9A: On the *left*, the fat cell and its receptors in a *female* shows a ratio of 7:1. (Alpha to Beta Receptors)

G. 9B: On the *right*, a fat cell and Its receptors has a *male* ratio of 1:1. (1 Alpha to 1 Beta Receptor)

of connective tissues to hold the skin and fat cells in their normal positions.

3. Fat cells from the waist down have a greater ratio of alpha receptors (fat storing) to beta receptors (fat burning). The ratio is approximately one beta receptor for every five alpha receptors.

4. The connective tissue layers in men are different from women's. Men's connective tissues overlap in a crisscross fashion; women's don't.

This is why cellulite occurs mainly on the "saddle bag" area, around the knees and on the buttocks, and why it seems to be almost indestructible. This is why generations of women believed that once cellulite made its ugly appearance, they were doomed to live with it for the rest of their lives. Cellulite is not something that can be treated by over-the-counter remedies and lifestyle alterations. Historically, there have been numerous remedies that have consistently failed. These include creams, lotions, massage machines, manual massage, diet and exercise. See Figure 10.

In the next chapter, you'll learn about the process whereby cellulite forms, as well as how certain factors can make the problem worse. ◊

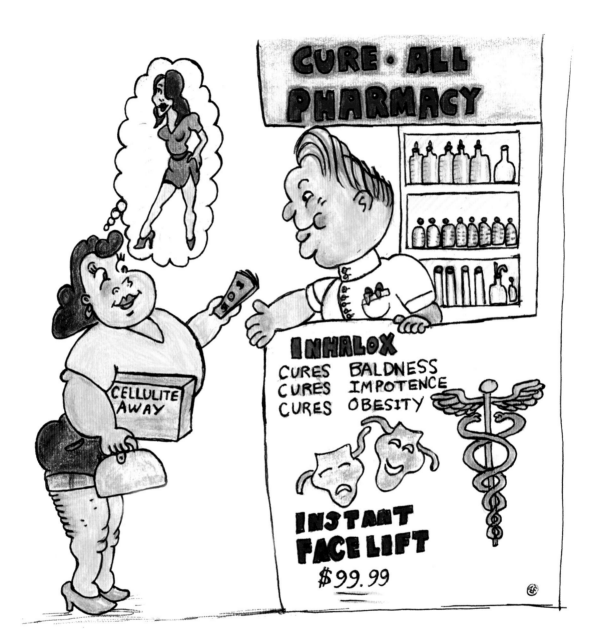

Fig. 10: Cellulina buys an anti-cellulite kit...

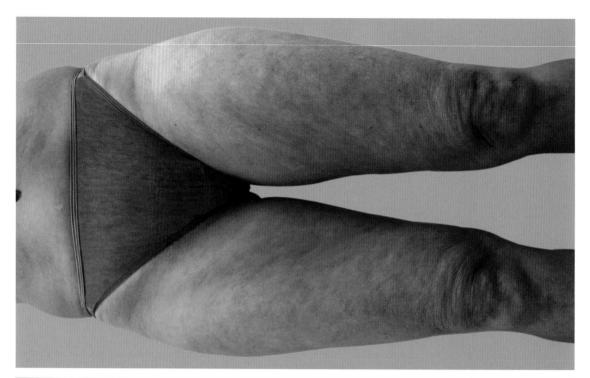

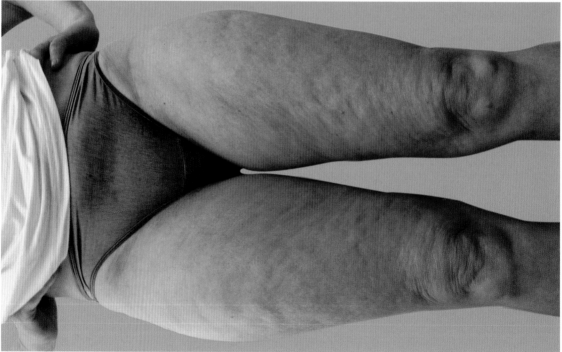

FIG. 11A-11B This is a woman who swims three hours a day for approximately five to six days a week. She was treated with 12 sessions of Mesotherapy. She also used Mesolysis™ Cellulite cream in conjunction with the treatments. The bottom photo is *before*. *Top* is *after*.

Lionel Bissoon

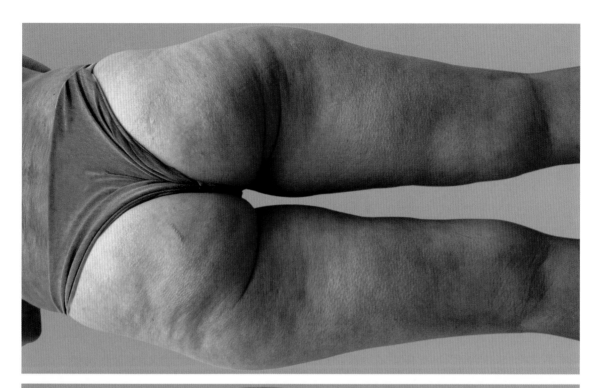

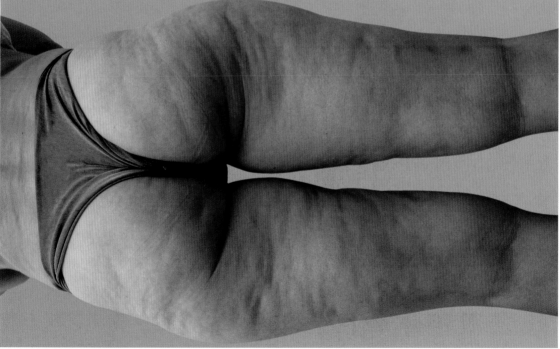

Fig. 12A-12B This is the same woman.

Lionel Bissoon

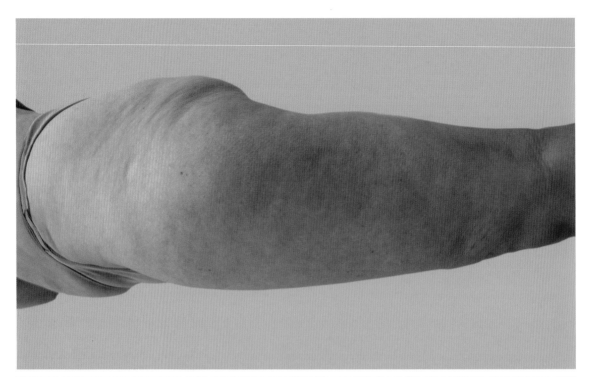

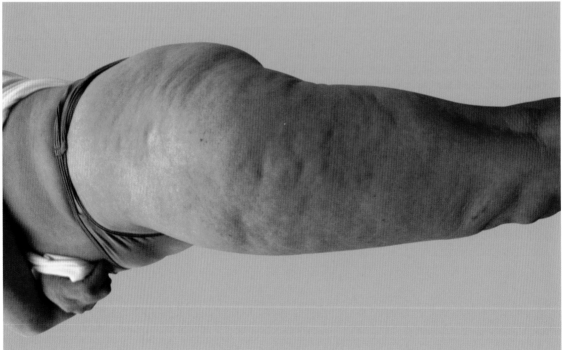

Fig. 13A-13B This is the same woman. The large, deep dimple in the upper aspect of the thigh that is seen in the "*Before*" photo was treated with Subcision™. (The *top* photo shows the *after* effects.)

Lionel Bissoon

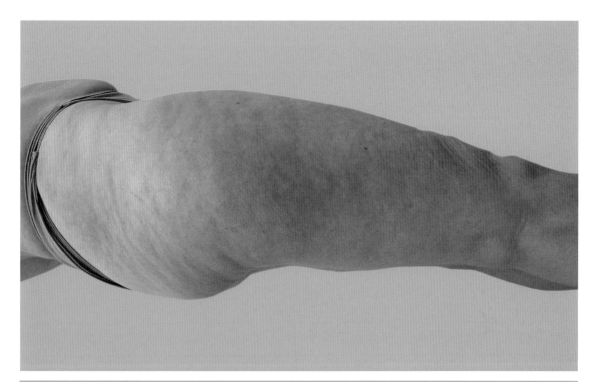

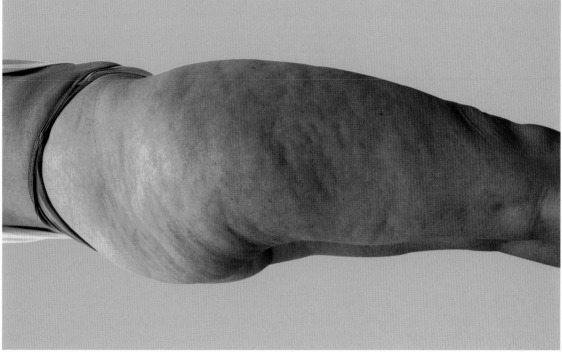

FIG. **14A-14B** The same woman

Lionel Bissoon

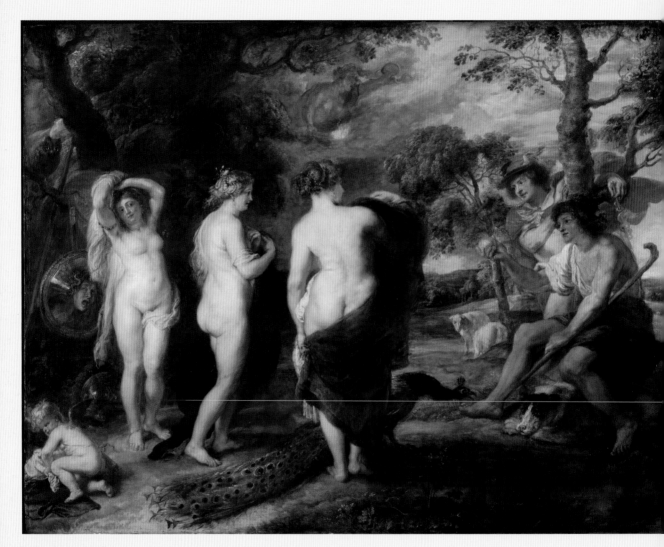

FIG. 1: "The Judgment of Paris," by Peter Paul Rubens

© National Gallery, London

3. *Cellulite Facts and* Fictions

The term "cellulite" was first coined around 1923 by

the French author Alquier. The appearance of little

cellular nodules probably inspired the term, because the

skin comes to resemble a collection of large cells

pushing against the skin, causing a ruffled appearance.

Another synonym for cellulite is "riding breeches."

While French physicians often refer to *riding breeches,*

English speakers use the term "saddlebags" to describe

fat deposits over the female hips that are sometimes

synonymous with cellulite.

But what is cellulite, and how does it form?

By definition, cellulite is a disease, but it is treated as a cosmetic medical condition—one characterized by unsightly dimpling of the skin on the hips, thighs and buttocks. The condition affects women of all shapes, sizes and ages. If you like medical jargon, the technical terms for cellulite are "adiposis edematosa" or "lipodystrophy," which describe the abnormal appearance of fat cells caused by poor circulation and lymph drainage, resulting in the degeneration of connective tissues that hold fat and skin cells in the normal position. That's the condensed version of the "domino effect of damage."

In my opinion, neither of these terms correctly describes the condition. The former suggests that there is fluid accumulation in the fatty tissues, while the latter attributes cellulite to dysfunctional fatty tissue.

Not every disease requires a fancy Latin name. The term cellulite adequately describes the problem. When you use the word "cellulite," everyone knows what you mean. Many authors do not conceive of cellulite as a disease. In fact, cellulite is a disease associated with aging, caused by changes in the body's biochemistry, physiology and anatomy. When such changes negatively affect the heart and other internal organs, we give them fancy names and diagnostic codes. Cellulite belongs in the same category.

Cellulite as a Disability

Because it's thought of as a cosmetic problem, the mainstream medical profession has paid little attention to the causes of cellulite, and hasn't pursued treatment options very aggressively. Ninety-nine percent of physicians probably don't know how to examine and grade cellulite. This is not taught in medical school and residency. Plastic surgeons and dermatologists are considered skin "gurus," but they cannot examine, grade and treat cellulite.

Plastic surgeons and dermatologists often advise patients that there is no treatment. They have adopted a "why bother?" attitude.

Plastic surgeons and dermatologists often advise patients that there is no treatment. They have adopted a "why bother?" attitude. In fact, in 2004, the American Academy of Dermatology fought against a presentation on cellulite by Dr. Mitchell Goldman at their annual national convention. Dr. Goldman is quoted as saying, "American Dermatologists have been ignoring cellulite, but they need to start paying attention." He goes on to say, "Patients are asking questions because the press is talking. If they can't go to a dermatologist for answers, where will they go?"★

I had a patient whose husband is a surgeon. He convinced her that there is no treatment for cellulite, and she should stop her foolish quest. Although she was emotionally devastated, she listened to the "brilliant" doctor—a man who is supposed to care about patients, but convinced his own wife that she should live with an emotional and physical disability rather than seek help. This is often the case with mainstream medicine. Physicians have the attitude of, "If I don't know about it, it must not be good." Someone once told Christopher Columbus that he would fall off the edge of the Earth if he sailed too far. This is the attitude of some modern physicians who are allegedly "steeped in scientific knowledge."

Dr. Irwin Gonzalez, former Department Chairman of Physical Medicine and Rehabilitation at Beth Israel, New York, described a disability as the following: "The inability to do something, which you previously did effortlessly without thinking about it." For this reason, I classify cellulite as a disability, not a cosmetic problem. See Figure 2.

It qualifies as a disability because the condition can prevent women from leading normal, active, satisfying lives. Now wait… don't rush to the DMV to apply for special license plates or start parking in handicapped zones. I'm simply saying what most of you already know. Women with cellulite often experience

I classify cellulite as a disability, not just a cosmetic problem. It qualifies as a disability because the condition can prevent women from leading normal, active, satisfying lives.

★ *"Solving the Cellulite Puzzle," by Rebecca Bryant* Dermatology Times *January 1, 2005, www.DermatologyTimes.com.*

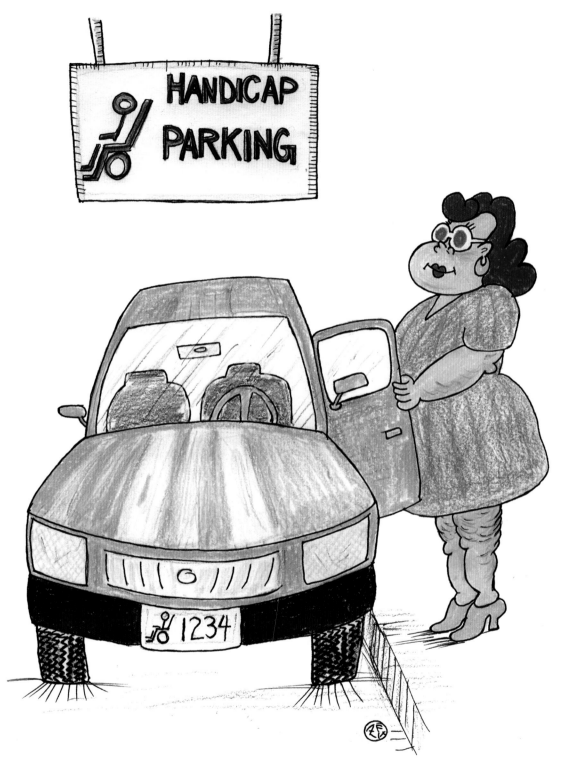

Fig. 2: "...for this reason, I classify cellulite as a disability, not a cosmetic problem."

CELLULITE'S EMOTIONAL AND PHYSICAL TOLL

Lowers self-esteem

Fear of ridicule and embarrassment

Affects romantic relationships and libido

Avoidance or decreased enjoyment of certain activities

Stress from continual efforts to hide or cover up cellulite

Time and money wasted on so-called "Cures"

Fig. 3

psychological distress, and suffer from diminished self-esteem. This negatively impacts their quality of life and their ability to function normally—the very definition of disability. See Figure 3.

Many women with cellulite complain that they feel uncomfortable wearing shorts, short skirts and swimsuits, and don't want loved ones (boyfriends, husbands, significant others) see them naked or see their legs. Often, they are reluctant to engage in sports and outdoor activities. In addition, these women usually have serious issues with body image. Given the "Hollywood Ideal" with which we're continuously bombarded, it's no wonder women with cellulite perceive themselves as unattractive, imperfect and flawed. It's no wonder they're afraid or ashamed to expose their bodies. They believe friends, family and loved ones will judge them and laugh at them. They worry their spouses will lose sexual interest. They hate explaining to their children "why mommy has holes in her legs."

Ironically, many celebrities and other "role models" have cellulite. They simply have access to special makeup, skilled photographers, photo editors and lighting designers. I have personally treated a number of entertainers with cellulite.

Kara is a 35-year-old administrative assistant from New Jersey whose cellulite appeared on her upper thighs when she was just 25. "Because of the severity of my cellulite, I never wore a bathing suit without some type of cover-up for my thighs. I was very self-conscious…and often would not walk in front of my boyfriend without some type of robe or cover-up. I love the beach, but I wouldn't go to the beach with him. I often dressed in longer, less fashionable clothes just because of my cellulite. No matter what I tried, including diet and exercise, creams and a machine method called *endermologie* nothing helped my condition.

I was often too embarrassed to talk to anyone about my problem with cellulite, and when I did talk about it with close friends, it was usually in a joking manner. I was too embarrassed to talk to anyone about it openly and to let anyone see how horrible it often made me feel."

Carol, a 27-year-old teacher from New York, developed cellulite on the backs of her legs and buttocks when she was 16. "I would never, ever wear shorts or allow the backs of my legs to be seen. If I was lying out in a bikini, I would never stand up or walk around without first putting a wrap around myself to cover up. I always thought that when [people] looked at me from behind, they would be disgusted and leave. So, I tried to make sure nobody saw me from behind. I tried dieting, exercising, liposuction and endermologie, but all these treatments failed— the cellulite remained.

I would discuss it [cellulite] with my friends, and they knew how insecure I was, but all they could do was try to make me feel better." (Their attempts did little to cheer her up.)

These are just some of the complaints I've repeatedly heard from women that I've successfully treated in my New York-California-Florida practice. Cellulite may not affect women's careers or their daily workplace routines, but it certainly tarnishes their social and emotional lives. We live in a society where quality of life is a big issue, and women with cellulite frequently complain about the condition's impact on their lives. Sure, nobody has ever died from cellulite, but cellulite does have a serious, negative impact—physically and mentally.

Myth Busted

Believe it or not, cellulite is more prominent in thin women. Rubenesque women have larger bone structures that seem to provide more "room for growth," if you will. Even as their fat cells grow larger, these women still seem to "wear" the extra weight well.

"I'm 42 years old, slim and tall," says Carmen of Westlake Village, California. My weight never goes past 116 pounds—aside from when I was pregnant. I don't have a model's body, but I work out, and I've worn thong underwear for the past 10 years. In other words, I was following Dr. Bissoon's lifestyle recommendations even before I met him, but I'm just prone to really bad cellulite.

I love the beach, but thanks to cellulite, I never wore anything clingy—no bikini bottoms. My 12-year-old daughter said it really embarrassed her when I wore clothes into the pool. After undergoing Mesotherapy, I have no large or dimpled cellulite anymore. I started wearing short shorts and miniskirts again. I'm going to start wearing a bikini. Now when my kids ask me to come in the water, I won't worry."

It's actually rare to see severe cellulite in women who are obese or seriously overweight. On the other hand, thin women seem to have less space available to nicely accommodate those fat cells as they grow. Therefore, when the connective tissue surrounding the fat chambers ("septae") becomes weakened, fat cells herniate through the subcutaneous layer, causing cellulite to appear.

The worst cellulite I've seen in my five years as a Mesotherapist appeared in thin women. Interestingly, obese women usually don't complain to me about cellulite. Their biggest issue usually involves a desire to lose weight, whereas thinner women are more concerned with eliminating cellulite.

Cellulite Season

Beginning in April, cellulite becomes a media issue, since every women's magazine is compelled to write a "timely" story on this intractable problem. Most stories lack any substance, and simply repeat the very same (bad) advice. The reason? Most writers turn to dermatologists and plastic surgeons as their sources. Often, these "experts" speak like trained parrots—spewing the same tired phrases ad nauseam: "there is nothing to do," "just live with it," "try diet and exercise." See Figure 4.

These two groups of physicians probably know nothing about diet and exercise, but keep regurgitating what they have always been told.

Don't let these nay-sayers dictate your health and well-being!

Cellulite takes years to develop, and cannot be cured between May and July. If there is to be a "cellulite season," let it be September through May. This is a better time to receive treatment than the height of swimsuit season. See Figure 5.

Cellulite Formation

In my theory of cellulite formation, cellulite is first triggered by a decrease in circulating estrogens. See Figure 6. Estrogen levels

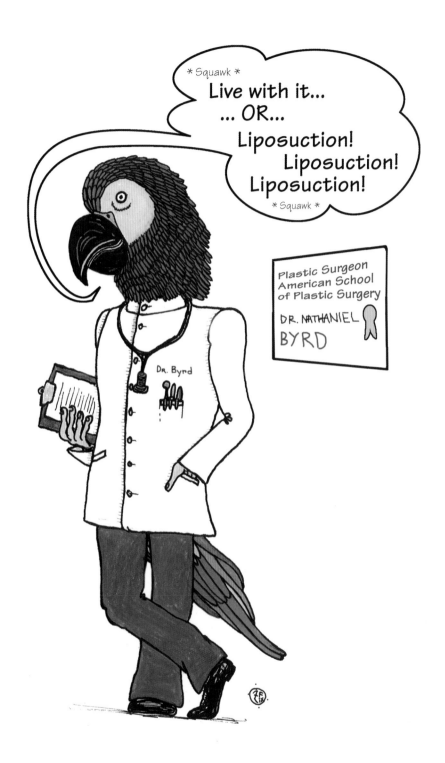

Fᴵɢ. 4: Dr. Byrd articulates the view of cellulite held by plastic surgeons and dermatologists.

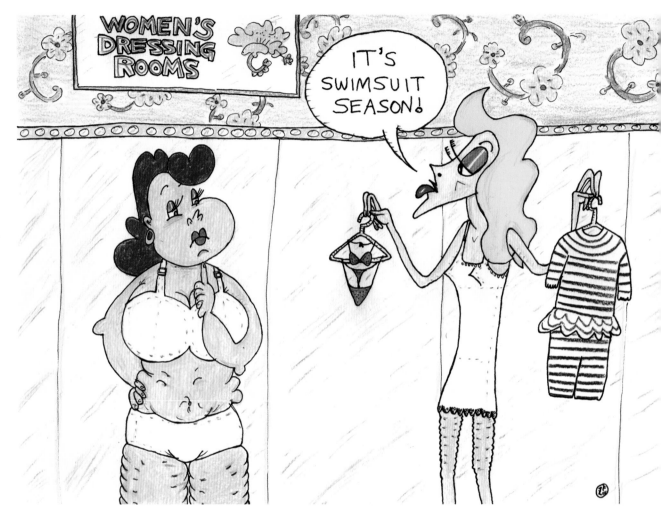

FIG. 5: Cellulina and Ana Rexia go shopping for bathing suits...

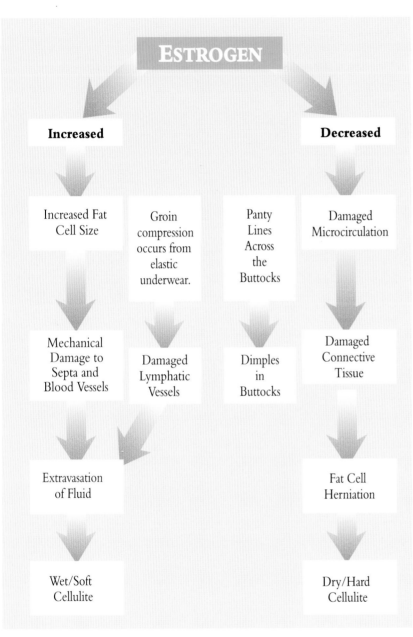

ESTROGEN

Increased

Increased Fat Cell Size	Groin compression occurs from elastic underwear.	Panty Lines Across the Buttocks	Damaged Microcirculation
Mechanical Damage to Septa and Blood Vessels	Damaged Lymphatic Vessels	Dimples in Buttocks	Damaged Connective Tissue
Extravasation of Fluid			Fat Cell Herniation
Wet/Soft Cellulite			Dry/Hard Cellulite

Decreased

FIG. 6: Factors Involved in Cellulite Formation

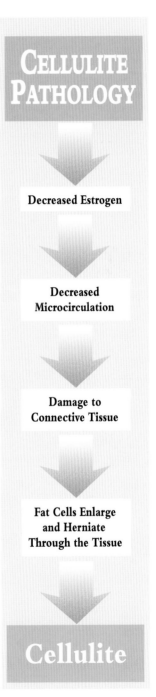

CELLULITE PATHOLOGY

Decreased Estrogen

Decreased Microcirculation

Damage to Connective Tissue

Fat Cells Enlarge and Herniate Through the Tissue

Cellulite

FIG. 7: Effects of Estrogen on Cellulite

usually begin to decrease in women aged 25 to 35. As estrogen levels slowly decrease, this affects the microscopic blood vessels carrying oxygen and nutrients to the fat cells, connective tissues and the supporting structure of the fat cells. Once this hormonal decline occurs, blood vessels become more *fibrotic*, which means they become more brittle. They also become sclerotic or hardened. The diameter of the blood vessels thus becomes narrower, the vessels harden, and they become leaky. The result is a decreased flow of blood and nutrients to the fall cells, connective tissue and the dermis in general. Another result is that depleted cellular nutrients build up as toxic waste matter in the tissues of the thighs, hips and buttocks. This waste material causes inflammation and eventually free radical damage. *Free radicals, or highly reactive oxygen derivatives, are released from immune cells in an attempt to clean and re-build the area.*

Lower levels of nutrients and oxygen available to the tissues in the area of incipient cellulite formation lead to decreased secretion activity from "fibroblasts," the cells responsible for repairing the septae (a band of connective tissue, composed of collagen, that surrounds the fat chambers). When the fibroblasts do not secrete sufficient collagen to maintain septae thickness, the septae thin and weaken and develop microscopic holes.

The next domino to fall involves the fat cells, which become "hypertrophied"—larger. As they enlarge, the fat cells herniate or rupture through the holes in the septae. Fat cell herniation produces the cottage cheese or orange peel effects of the skin.

To summarize the steps involved in cellulite formation: cellulite is caused by a decrease in estrogen, which leads to decreased microcirculation of the blood and lymph, and decreased secretion activity from fibroblasts. A build-up of waste materials in your tissues causes inflammation and gradual weakening of connective tissue though which the fat cells

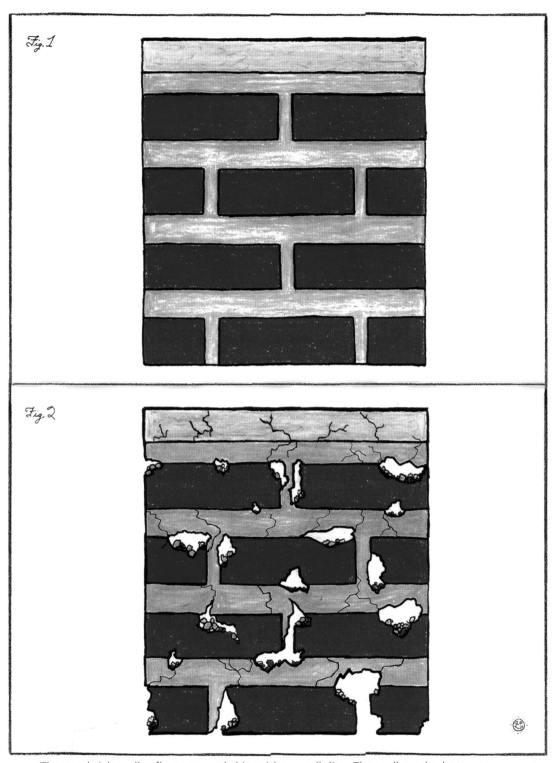

FIG. 8: The top brick wall reflects normal skin without cellulite. The wall on the bottom represents what happens as cellulite develops.

herniate. The skin becomes distorted—with the subsequent appearance of cottage cheese, orange peel or mattress appearance on the skin lying above the process. See Figure 7.

You can also think of it this way: in the dermis, the fat chambers (or lobes) are arranged like bricks in a wall, with the septae comprising the mortar between the bricks. Under normal conditions, the bricks are well stacked and create the appearance of a smooth, flat surface. When cellulite develops, some of the bricks appear to have been stacked too far forward or backward in the wall, and the mortar starts to crack and collapse. See Figure 8.

Lymphatic Troubles

Lymphatic vessels are very important in cellulite formation. Normally, these vessels efficiently drain fluids in the tissues back into the veins, which eventually carry the tissue fluids back to the heart. The deterioration of the lymphatic vessels is a three-stage process involving: Stage One Passive Congestion, where lymph fluids fail to drain from the surrounding tissue. Stage Two occurs when lymphatic fluids actually begin to leak out of the lymphatic capillaries. This brings us to Stage Three, when damage to the surrounding tissue commences.

I have described my theory of cellulite evolution based upon the available literature and observations of patients. Although other physicians who have studied and/or treated cellulite agree on most points, there isn't total unanimity on all of the details in the processes that cause cellulite. However, as you'll see in Chapter 4, I have successfully treated hundreds of cellulite sufferers by premising my approach and methods on the theory presented herein. I believe that my success provides at least indirect evidence of my theory's validity. I am not aware of any other physician who has examined and treated cellulite on a daily basis during the last five years, as intently as myself. Understanding and curing cellulite is my passion. I am dedicated to improving the physical and mental health of my patients.

Hard and Soft Cellulite

Occasionally, you'll see references to "soft cellulite" vs. "hard cellulite." Here's the difference: the soft variety involves cases where lymph fluid build-up in the underlying tissues is so significant that the superficial skin has a wet, boggy feeling to it. The retained fluid imparts a soft appearance to the cellulite. "Hard" cellulite is so called because there is little or no lymphatic fluid accumulation. The lymphatic vessels are doing their job of draining away fluid, and hence, there is no fluid build-up within the tissues.

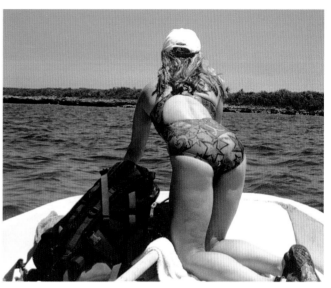

Fig. 9: This photo shows a competitive swimmer who was training for a minimum of three hours a day, yet she has a cottage cheese appearance to her legs.

Lionel Bissoon

In other words, soft cellulite is caused by lymphatic problems. Treating such cellulite is difficult because there is usually overlying loose skin associated with the condition. Merely draining the accumulated fluids will leave behind extra amounts of loose skin.

Functional Cellulite

This is a category of my own creation, and it is based on hundreds of patient evaluations. Women who complain about cellulite *only* when they are sitting (especially with legs crossed), or when standing in certain positions are often describing *functional cellulite*. What is actually happening in this type of cellulite is that the aforementioned activities cause compression of the underlying muscles, producing tension on the collagen fibers connecting the muscle to the skin. This causes the

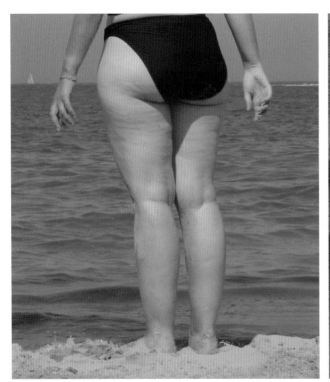
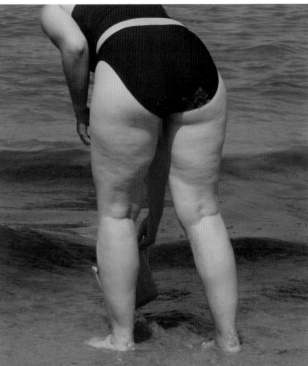
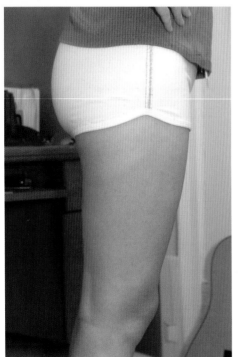
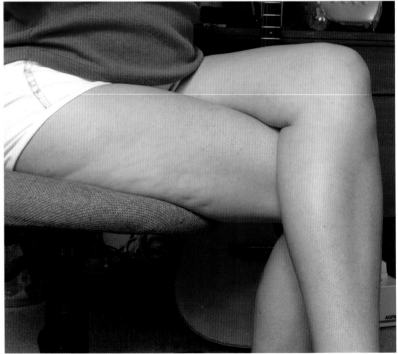

FIG. 10A-10D: Figures A and B show a woman at the beach standing, and then bending forward. This motion increased the appearance of cellulite. Photo C and D shows a 33 year old female with cellulite appearing while sitting. The above photos are examples of *functional* cellulite.

Lionel Bissoon

63 • Cellulite Facts and Fictions

appearance of cellulite on the muscle tension, which disappears when the tension is removed. This type of cellulite can make any grade of cellulite appear more severe. Often times, the media will print photographs of celebrities indulging in different activities or sitting in certain positions which portray dimpling of the skin. See Figure 10A-D.

Diet and Exercise?

It is commonly thought that poor diet and lack of exercise cause cellulite, and that a healthier diet and increased exercise will reduce or eliminate the condition. Based on my observations and reviews of the published literature, there is some connection between cellulite, diet and exercise, but not a direct one. Although a healthier lifestyle can reduce the appearance of cellulite, it's *not* a real or effective treatment. Connective tissues behave like an accordion. See Figure 11A-B. When your weight decreases, the tissues collapse onto each other; when you gain weight, the tissues expand to display visible cellulite. I treat many female athletes and personal trainers who engage in vigorous physical activities five to seven days a week. Refer back to Figure 10. They still have cellulite. Given this, how can anyone claim that diet and exercise alone are the ultimate solution? Some dermatologists and plastic surgeons make this claim—yet these physicians have absolutely no training in diet and exercise. As a physician trained in Physiatry, I have treated sports injuries for many years. I believe I write with some authority on this topic.

Of course, a sedentary lifestyle centered on the consumption of junk food certainly doesn't help the problem. A high caloric intake, combined with a sedentary lifestyle, results in fat deposition. Remember, it's easier to store fat from the waist down, because your body contains more alpha receptors in that region (seven alphas for every single beta) per fat cell,* as well as more

---

* *Alpha receptors, when stimulated, will make and store fat. Beta receptors will break down fat when stimulated.*

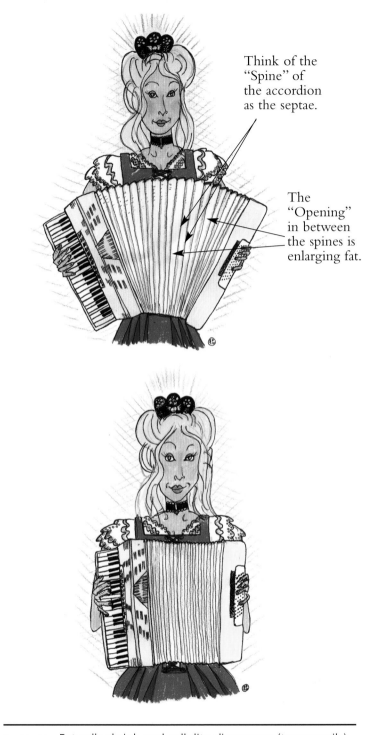

Think of the "Spine" of the accordion as the septae.

The "Opening" in between the spines is enlarging fat.

FIG. 11A-11B: Fat cells shrink and cellulite disappears (temporarily).

fat layers than men. Alpha and beta receptors are like microscopic antennae on the surface of fat cells. The antennae respond to signals received from the surrounding fluids and neighboring cells. Among those signals are hormone molecules, surface molecules such as fatty acids, carbohydrates, alcohol, pesticides, insecticides and toxic waste products, along with molecules present on neighboring cells. Plastic surgeons and dermatologists won't explain this concept to you, either because they honestly don't know or don't want to take the time. It is well established that infrequent use of your muscles decreases the pumping action exerted on the veins and lymphatic vessels.

The problem with dieting to cure already established cellulite is this: once cellulite erupts, your fat cells are already enlarged and the connective tissue has been damaged. Certain exercises and diets may shrink the fat cells, and cause tissues to collapse and compress upon themselves, giving the skin the temporary appearance of a normal texture. However, the moment the weight comes back, the cellulite comes back. Once again, your fat cells will enlarge and herniate through damaged connective tissues that were never repaired—and cannot be repaired with diet and exercise alone. Despite this, there are numerous anti-cellulite diets and exercise programs touted at any given time—just read any woman's magazine.

A number of women have complained to me, "Look doctor, I've gone on this diet, I've done these exercises, and the cellulite disappeared. But the moment I gained two pounds, the damned cellulite came back with a vengeance!"

I call this the "Accordion Effect." (Refer back to Figures 11A-B.) Don't succumb to the lure of any anti-cellulite diet: inevitably, you will be disappointed. Diets temporarily treat only one aspect of cellulite formation.

Diet and exercise do not change the underlying structure of the cellulite.

Diet and exercise do *not* change the underlying structure of the cellulite. All one can hope for in some cases is a decrease in the size of the fat cells. Nothing is done to repair the damaged collagen; nothing is done to increase localized circulation. Only Mesotherapy and Mesotherapy Stringcision™ in combination with certain lifestyle changes can make a difference. Lifestyle changes alone will not cure the condition, and often few visible changes in the appearance of cellulite occur. Historically, there have been numerous anti-cellulite programs based on diet and exercise, but none of them address the problem. Instead, they target the symptoms.

Creams and lotions have been around for decades, but none have worked, because creams and lotions do not penetrate the skin. They sit on the skin, and do nothing to affect the underlying pathology of the cellulite. Another advantage of Mesotherapy is that you'll want to schedule an annual follow-up session to maintain your legs.

Kara tried nearly every "cellulite cure" ever marketed. "I tried endermologie, and didn't see any noticeable results. I also tried just about every anti-cellulite cream on the market, and I even bought a handheld thigh massager. Before having Mesotherapy, I didn't see any improvement with my cellulite no matter what I tried."

Some people believe that deep and/or mechanical massage can break up the nodular appearance of herniated fat cells. However, the process can be extremely painful and often requires multiple treatments. The biggest problem with massage involves the inability of any massage therapist to apply consistent pressure to the skin. The pressure exerted varies throughout the day, and it varies on the number of patients he/she has worked with. Consistent application of pressure is simply impossible. Mechanical massage seeks to remedy this problem, but many women complain that it does nothing to improve cellulite.

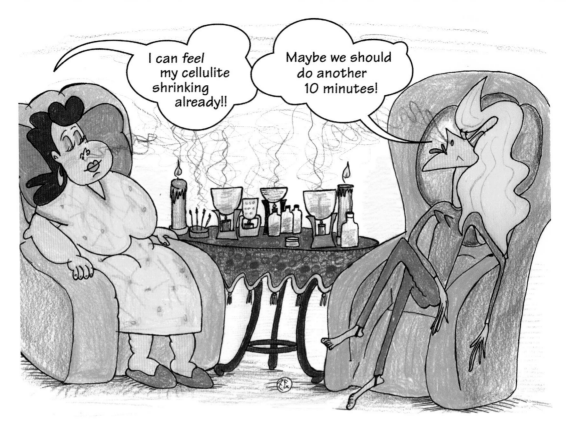

FIG. 12: Cellulina and Ana Rexia try Aromatherapy as a cellulite treatment...

Worse, it sometimes causes decreased elasticity of the skin—i.e., it makes the skin looser. Numerous women have complained to me of "loose skin" after a series of mechanical massages. It is probable such a deep massage destroys the integrity of the underlying connective and supportive tissues.

Another so-called cellulite solution involves aromatherapy. To the best of my knowledge, aromatherapy has absolutely no impact on cellulite. At most, the pleasing smells may enhance your mood during the session. You can't sniff your way to a cure. See Figure 12.

Although dieting does little to ameliorate cellulite, a diet rich in organic foods may help prevent the condition in the first place. As noted earlier, I believe that cellulite is largely a phenomenon that affects women in industrialized societies. This is based on my

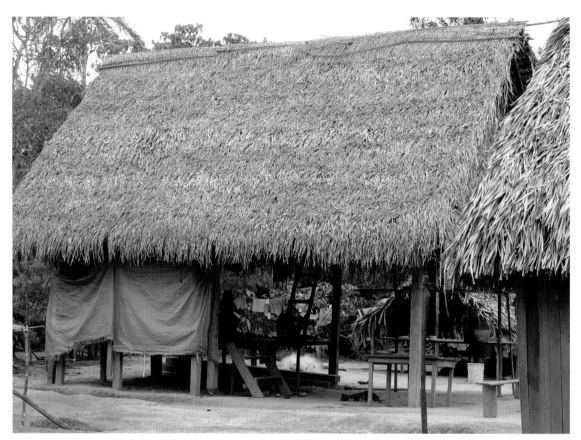

Fig. 13: This is a Shipibo Indian home in the Amazon.

Lionel Bissoon

observations of women in developing countries—especially those who live in "primitive" rural communities. I have often journeyed to a small village in Peru to assist the native peoples. I observed that women who live in the small "jungle towns" of South America eat much more organic food than their U.S. counterparts. In particular, they consume large quantities of plants in the yam/yucca family, which contain plenty of phyto-estrogens. These plant estrogens mimic the effects of naturally occurring estrogens in the body. So older women in these areas are, in effect, taking naturally occurring estrogen supplements that replace the decreasing hormone levels in their bodies.

In some cultures, there is also more consumption of soybeans and soybean products, which also contains estrogen-like products.

The observations of decreased cellulite among native peoples tends to support my argument that declining estrogen level is the main culprit in cellulite formation. The decrease in circulating estrogens causes a cascade of effects. In addition to promoting cellulite, decreased estrogen also plays a role in skin aging. Many scientific journals have published articles about the effects of decreased estrogen on skin aging, but none have addressed the effects of decreasing estrogen on cellulite formation.

In addition to eating organic foods, women in "developing" countries often walk a great deal, work in the fields, and—in general—lead a less sedentary lifestyle than American women. Their work consists of hard labor, which requires walking, carrying heavy loads, caring for children and maintaining their households—without all of the modern appliances available in Europe and North America. Even if they had vacuum cleaners and disposable floor mops, try keeping your house clean when the roof is made from thatch, the walls from mud and the floors from packed soil. See Figure 13.

Yes, diet and exercise may play a role. But they seem to play a role in preventing cellulite, not reducing or eliminating it once it occurs. Remember: these "Third World" women lead active lives almost from the day they're born. And, not only do they consume mostly organic food, they also tend to wear less restrictive clothing and undergarments. (More about clothing in Chapter 8.)

Of course, every "Third-World" country has its large metro-politan areas, and in the big cities, you will find women who recently migrated from smaller, rural communities. Invariably, many of these women develop cellulite. They consume more processed foods, their lifestyles become more sedentary, and they adopt more restrictive undergarments. Figure 13A-13D shows Shipibo rural women in their daily, non-sedentary lifestyle.

Female connective tissue has a radial appearance, whereas connective tissue in men has a cross-linked overlap appearance, making it stronger. That's the reason why men usually do not get cellulite.

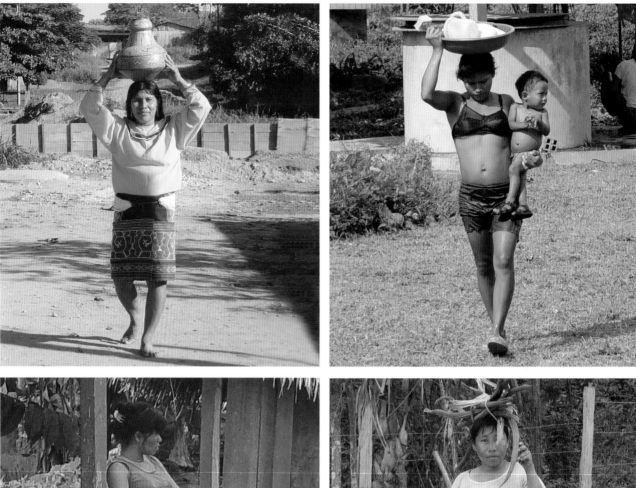
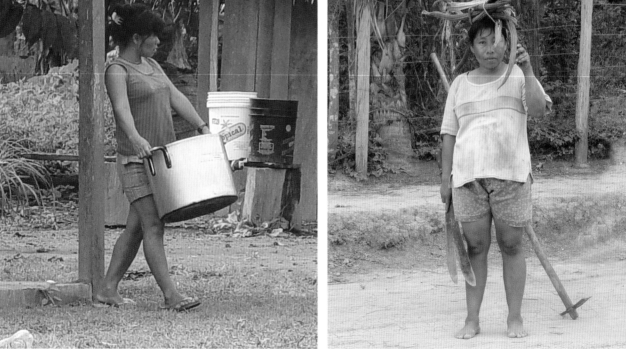

FIG. 14A-14D: Shipibo women of Peru are shown here in a typical day's work.

Lionel Bissoon

In sum, dieting and increased exercise may help reduce the appearance of cellulite after it's occurred, but do not repair the underlying problem. They do not mend damaged connective tissues that allow the fat cells to herniate.

Heredity

Heredity may, or may not, play a role in cellulite formation. Actually, medical science is almost certain that heredity does not play a role because such a large percentage of women develop cellulite (in the industrialized world). The condition is definitely determined by gender, because the underlying connective tissue in women is different from that in men. Female connective tissue has a radial appearance, whereas connective tissue in men has a cross-linked overlap appearance, making it stronger. That's the reason why men usually do not get cellulite.

Medications and other health conditions may play a role in the development of cellulite. For example, some women have noted weight gain caused by using pharmaceuticals such as prednisone. This weight gain could result in the destruction of the collagen connective tissues, which allows herniation of fat cells. Several patients undergoing infertility treatments have noticed development of cellulite after using the medication Lupron.

Pregnancy

Needless to say, pregnancy has a profound affect on a woman's body. And, because pregnancy can cause fluid retention and fat storage, it may lead to cellulite formation. During gestation, the uterus increases in size, pressing upon the lymph vessels and veins. This causes a reduction in lymph and blood drainage that triggers fluid retention in the tissues, and spurs development of cellulite. Of course, this situation is temporary. Immediately following birth, pressure on the draining vessels is relieved, and the flow returns to normal levels. In addition, pregnancy causes weight gain in the hips and buttocks, *in the areas where there are three fat pads. Remember, the subcutaneous layer of fat in the hips, buttocks and around the knees are hormone sensitive.* As the fat cells become larger, they exert pressure on the collagen fibers in the fat lobes, resulting in the destruction of the fat lobes. Cellulite caused by pregnancy is the best example of how cellulite occurs, since all of the formation mechanisms are working at this time.

During the period of limited drainage, however, lymphatic fluids accumulate in tissues, along with precipitated proteins and begin to form fibers. In addition, estrogen decreases and progesterone increases, causing the fat cells to enlarge around the legs, thighs and buttocks. It should be noted that during the first two trimesters, estrogen is low compared to progesterone, but high when compared to the non-pregnant state. In the third trimester, estrogen increases and peaks. As the fat cells grow, they exert pressure on the collagen and septum separating the fat lobes, resulting in destruction of the septae.

Although estrogen levels are low compared with progesterone during pregnancy, estrogen increases immediately before delivery while progesterone decreases. Many have proposed that cellulite is caused by high estrogen stemming from pregnancy. However, non-pregnant women almost never achieve these hormonal levels, so—in theory—they shouldn't develop cellulite. Others subscribe to high estrogen theories because estrogen increases the sensitivity of the alpha (fat-storing) receptors, producing enlarged fat cells that exert pressure on the septae, along with retained lymphatic fluids.

Although pregnancy is a temporary state, its side effects may trigger cellulite formation, even after the prerequisite hormonal conditions disappear following birth. Remember that once it's launched, cellulite formation becomes a vicious cycle.

Not every pregnant woman develops cellulite, thus proving that increased estrogen is not always the causative factor. If increased estrogen was truly the culprit, every woman taking birth control pills would have cellulite.

Dubious Malefactors

Liposuction. Kara underwent liposuction when she was 31. "I decided to get liposuction on my thighs, which worsened the condition. After liposuction, my thighs exhibited a much lumpier and dispersed cellulite formation."

Tina, a 46-year-old entrepreneur living in New Jersey, also complained that liposuction worsened her cellulite when she underwent the procedure seven years ago. "The doctor did a horrible job. I looked worse than I did before. The skin was extremely uneven, and it looked really bad."

These stories are not uncommon. Occasionally, you will read magazine articles about women who claim that liposuction exacerbated their cellulite. What these women are actually complaining about is the *appearance* of their cellulite, post-liposuction. When performing liposuction, physicians sometimes get too close to the skin, and remove a little too much fat. This may amplify—or cause the appearance—of new dimpling. In other words, liposuction may cause cellulite to look worse, but it hasn't actually caused the underlying condition to worsen. I realize that this is a fine distinction, so think of it this way: wearing clothing that's too small may cause you to *appear* fatter, but it doesn't actually *make* you fatter.

There is no evidence that liposuction, when performed correctly, has any affect on cellulite.

Liposuction may cause cellulite to look worse, but it hasn't actually caused the underlying condition to worsen.

Moreover, liposuction was never intended as a cellulite cure, because the fat cells responsible for cellulite occur in the subcutaneous fat layer, which is inaccessible for the purposes of liposuction.

Liposuction is a procedure for sculpting the body, not for treating cellulite. If your plastic surgeon or dermatologist recommends liposuction for cellulite, get another opinion. Your doctor is being unethical.

In addition, I have seen some post-liposuction patients who claim to have noticed a reduction in the appearance of cellulite. The cellulite was still present, but there was a decreased appearance.

Posture. I don't believe posture affects cellulite. However, there are instances when cellulite is more predominant on one side of the body. This is because the body is not completely symmetrical. We're all a little lopsided. Because some asymmetry is always present, I have noticed many instances where cellulite is more pronounced on the right leg vs. the left leg, and so forth. But posture doesn't really affect cellulite formation. However, some postures can exaggerate one's cellulite.

Stress. Neither do I believe that stress contributes to cellulite. On the other hand, pollution and free radicals do contribute to the problem. Tissue damage caused by free radical damage does foster destruction of both the underlying and overlying tissues. And environmental pollution contributes to cellulite in the sense that the air you breath becomes laden with chemicals that are toxic to the cells.

Temperature. There are some physicians who believe that moving from cold to warm climates during the winter months helps to facilitate the development of cellulite by causing the constriction and dilation of blood vessels. In other words, when

Taking estrogen will not cure cellulite, because damage to the connective tissue, decreased circulation, and herniated fat cells have already occurred.

you are exposed to cold temperatures, the vessels constrict, and when you enter a warm room, they become dilated. It is possible that temperature contributes to cellulite formation.

The Real Culprit

Once cellulite debuts on your thighs, buttocks or even the back of your knees, dieting and increased exercise can do little to remedy the condition. This is because decreasing estrogen level is the chief suspect in cellulite formation. Based on this supposition, and my discussion of how eating foods rich in naturally occurring estrogen-like products may help Third-World women prevent cellulite, you'd think that that the cure is pretty self-evident: Take estrogen supplements as prescribed by a doctor.

Unfortunately, this is a case where the "obvious solution" doesn't work. Taking estrogen will not cure cellulite, because damage to the connective tissue, decreased circulation and herniated fat cells have already occurred. Taking estrogen *will* retard cellulite development, but won't erase your *existing* dimpling.

At this point, some of you may be tired of reading the bad news, and anxious to learn about Mesotherapy—what it is and how it works to actually cure cellulite. If so, flip ahead to Chapter 5. If you can hold your horses, the next chapter allows you to gauge the severity of your cellulite and help you determine if you're an appropriate candidate for Mesotherapy.

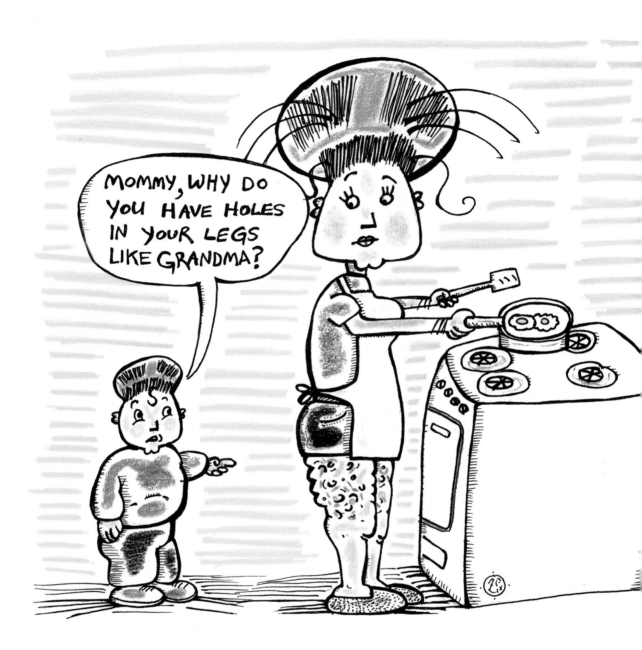

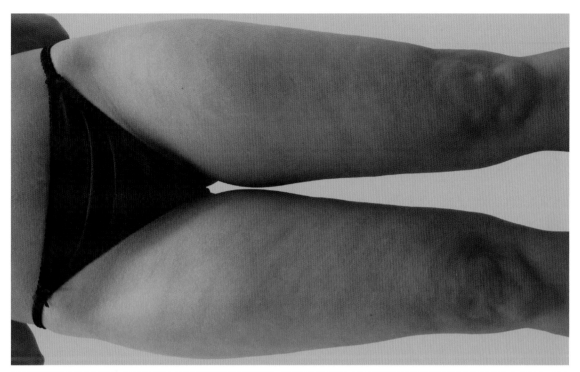

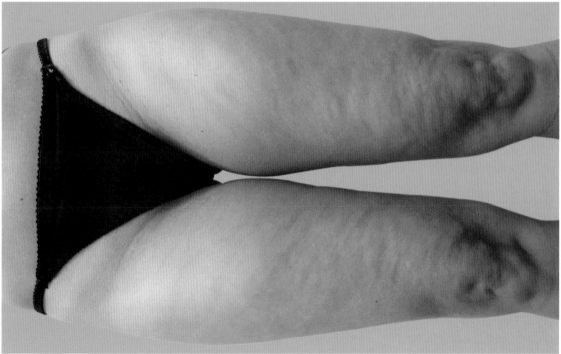

FIG. 15A-15B: This woman was treated with ten sessions of Mesotherapy and she used the Mesolysis™ Cellulite cream in conjunction with the treatments. The *bottom* photo is her *before.*

Lionel Bissoon

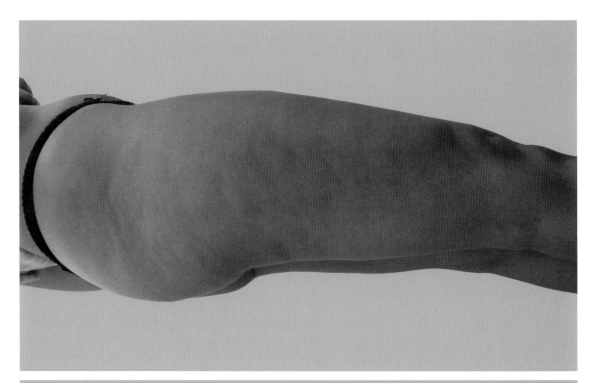

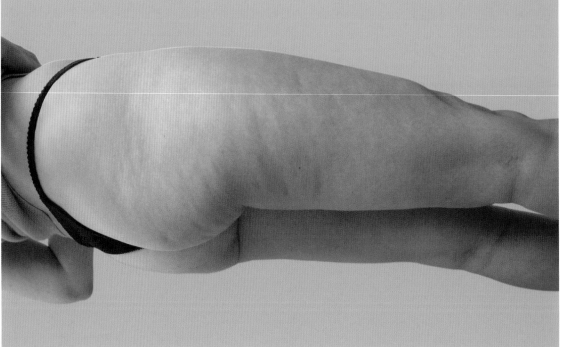

FIG. 16A-16B: This shows the same patient.

Lionel Bissoon

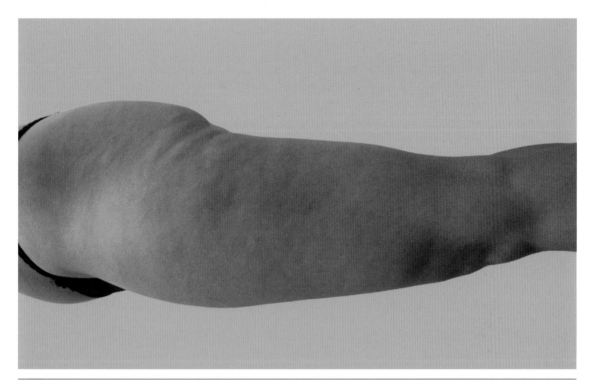

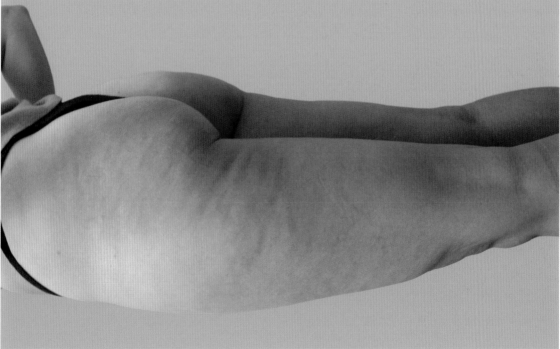

Fig. 17A-17B: This is the same patient.

Lionel Bissoon

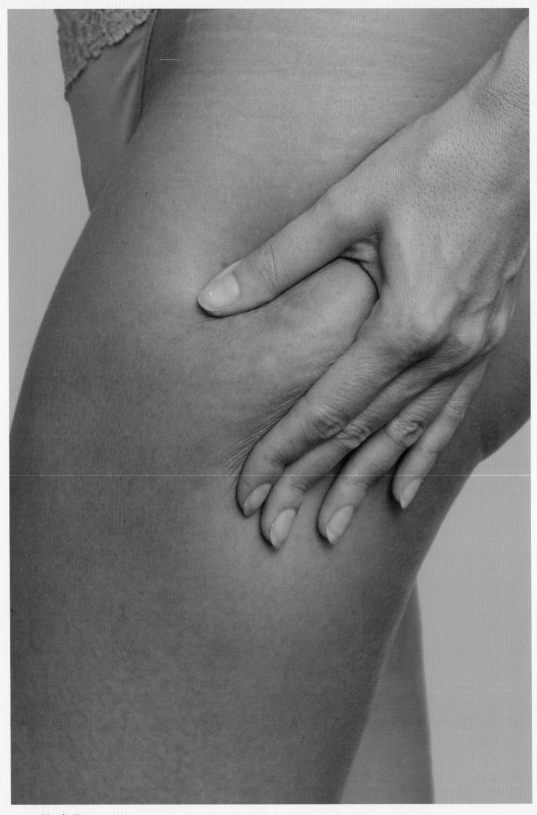

FIG. 1: Pinch Test

Lionel Bissoon

4. *Your Self*
Exam

Cellulite is classified according to the severity of its

appearance—its symptoms. While some women may

exhibit only a few rimples and dimples on the upper

thigh that are barely noticeable, some unfortunate

women manifest such extreme mattress effects that

the afflicted areas look as though they've gone through

a cheese grater. I use a cellulite classification system

that involves just four stages. There are other grading

systems, but this one is probably the simplest and

easiest tool for self-evaluation. Commonly referred to

as the Nurnberger System, (it was named after the

German scientist who performed one of the single

most important studies on cellulite), and has been

widely used since 1978. See Figure 2.

CLASSIFICATION OF CELLULITE

Stage 0	No visible cellulite while standing.
Stage 1	The skin is smooth while standing or lying down, but the Pinch Test produces a mattress appearance. See Figure 3A–5D.
Stage 2	Cottage cheese appearance to the skin is visible while standing. It disappears when laying down.
Stage 3	Mattress appearance is visible regardless of whether the woman is standing or lying down. See Figure 5A–5D.

FIG. 2

Even so, it's best to evaluate yourself—even if you think you've successfully escaped cellulite (so far). You may not have "cottage cheese" thighs. Maybe you simply have a few dimples on your buttocks. No need to worry, right? Well, dimples are symptomatic of cellulite and early intervention therapy is always best. You needn't have a cottage cheese appearance of the skin to be diagnosed with cellulite and begin therapy.

To use the "pinch test," hold your skin between the thumb and other fingers, lift and gradually apply pressure. This compresses the different structures of your skin, and creates a bulging of the upper fat-cell chamber system. This temporarily enhances the dimpling of the skin, allowing it to become more visible. Obviously, you don't want cellulite to be more visible all the time. However, this test helps you determine if cellulite is present, even if you've never noticed it during the course of daily activities. Needless to say, many women are unpleasantly surprised when they first perform the pinch test. See Figure 1.

Grade 3 is Hard to Treat

Here's another reason for self-diagnosis and early treatment. Although Mesotherapy can work near-miracles on women with Grade 1 or Grade 2 cellulite, Grade 3 may require a prolonged period of treatment. Women with borderline Grade 2 cellulite, or obvious Grade 2 cellulite, are the *ideal* candidates for Mesotherapy and Mesotherapy Stringcision™, as well as Subcision™ (See Chapter 6.)

I have treated women ages 21 to 68 for cellulite. However, if patients display Grade 3 cellulite, I advise them to carefully consider Mesotherapy because the number of treatment sessions can be very unpredictable, and therefore, expensive. Grade 3 cellulite requires a very long commitment from the patient, and is much, much harder to treat. I don't refuse to treat women with the severest cellulite. In deciding whether to treat Grade 3 cellulite, cost factors are a major consideration.

Non-Candidates for Mesotherapy

There are women whom I have refused to treat. In other cases, I have initially recommended that would-be patients reconsider the treatment—or at least mull the situation over—before deciding to commit time and money to the cure. This is not because I don't sympathize with the plight of cellulite sufferers. But there have been occasions when I have doubted whether the woman was motivated by a sincere desire to improve her appearance, or was coerced by loved ones and/or afflicted with a mental health problem.

Any cosmetic procedure—whether it's plastic surgery, liposuction or Mesotherapy—should be initiated *by* the patient, *for* the patient. Please, do not schedule an appointment with any Mesotherapist because you feel pressured by a boyfriend, husband or significant other. If you are completely uninterested in treating your cellulite via Mesotherapy, and your loved ones won't accept your decision, I'm afraid you're a candidate for "Dear Abby," and not Dr. Lionel Bissoon.

I will happily treat any woman who sincerely wants to eliminate unsightly dimples, ruffles and orange peel skin. I will turn away women whose loved ones have pushed them through my door. My program requires a big commitment. Someone who's been browbeaten into seeking treatment probably won't stick with the program for the long haul.

When I've encountered women seeking help because boyfriends or husbands pressured them into it, I've asked that they reconsider unless they truly believe that Mesotherapy will benefit *them* both physically and emotionally. Mesotherapy cures cellulite, not psycho-logical disorders and relationship problems.

I would also refuse—or even discontinue treatment—in cases where the patient insists on wearing the same kind of clothing, especially underwear, that contributes to cellulite formation. If they refuse to consider switching to cellulite-friendly undergarments, I would refuse to offer treatment. To do otherwise, would be like trying to swim up Niagara Falls, because the patient would be defeating whatever progress she made through Mesotherapy.

I'll talk more about undergarments and their relationship to cellulite in Chapter 8, where I will provide a detailed description of what Mesotherapy is, how it works, why it works and how the other treatment components that make up my program work together to help eradicate cellulite.

Some women have come to me complaining about cellulite, but my examinations revealed no evidence of cellulite. What I *have* discovered is redundant skin (loose skin) on the inner thighs and around the knees. Mesotherapy does not treat severe redundant

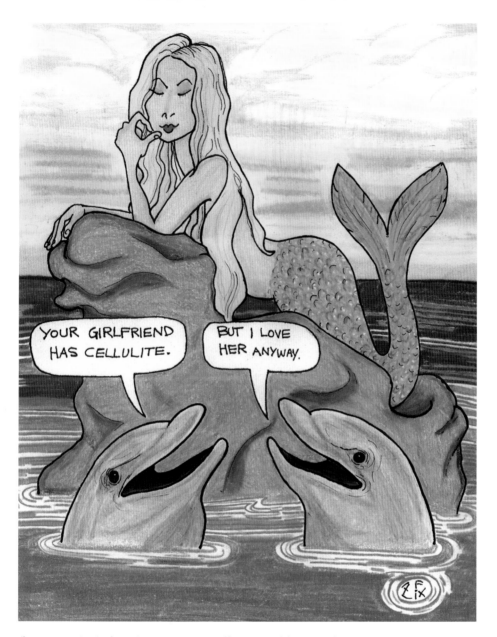

(loose sagging) skin. (However, it will treat mild to moderate redundant skin.) As this time, I suggest that these patients consult with a Board Certified cosmetic surgeon. The American Board of Cosmetic Surgery certifies physicians specializing in cosmetic surgery. Although thigh lifts are not common procedures, if you're considering one, consult with the ABCS to find a good surgeon. ◊

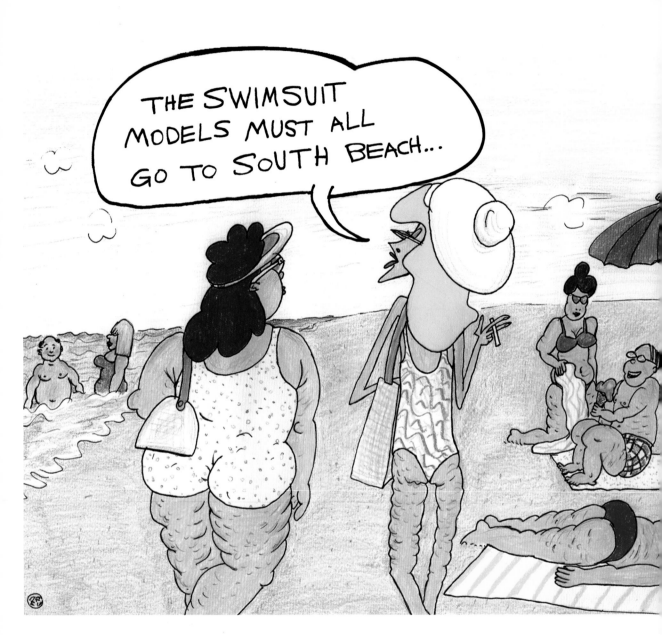

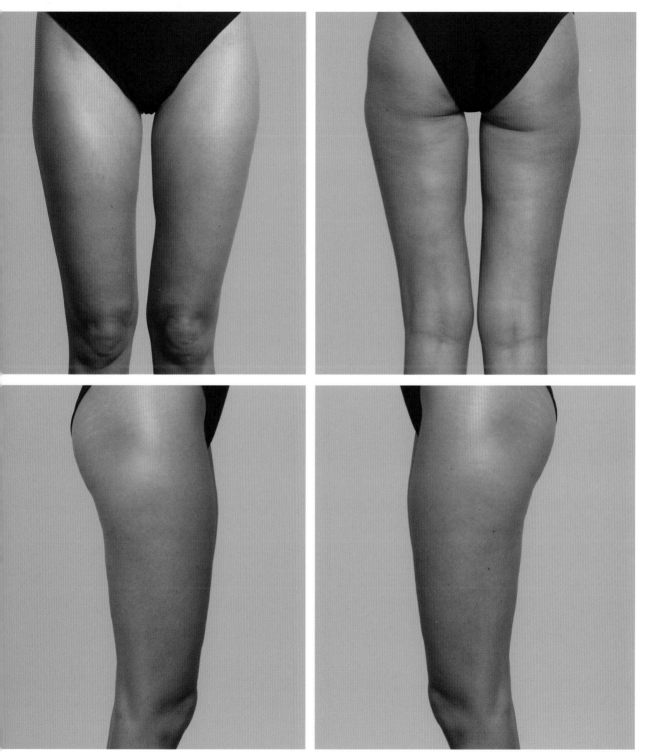

3A-3D: Woman Exhibiting Grade 1 Cellulite

Lionel Bissoon

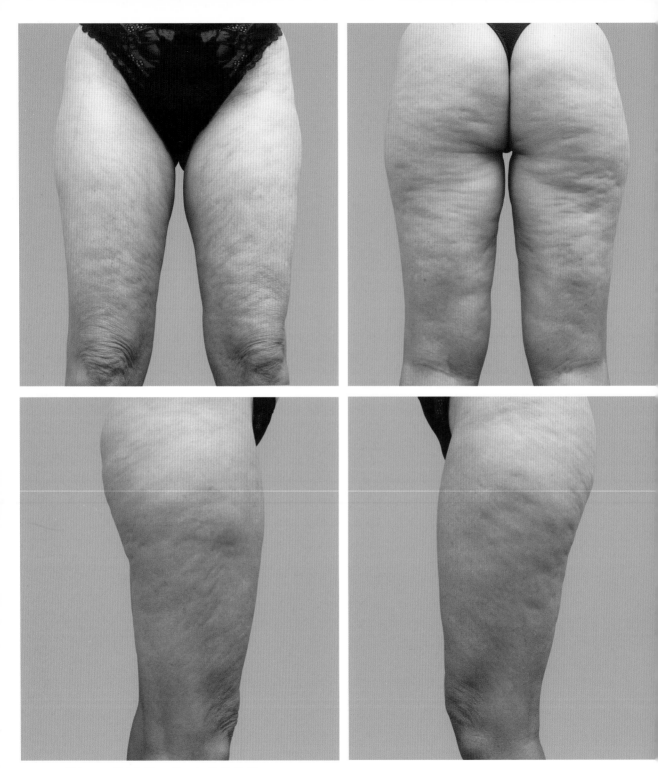

FIG. 4A-4D: Woman Exhibiting Grade 2 Cellulite

Lionel Bissoon

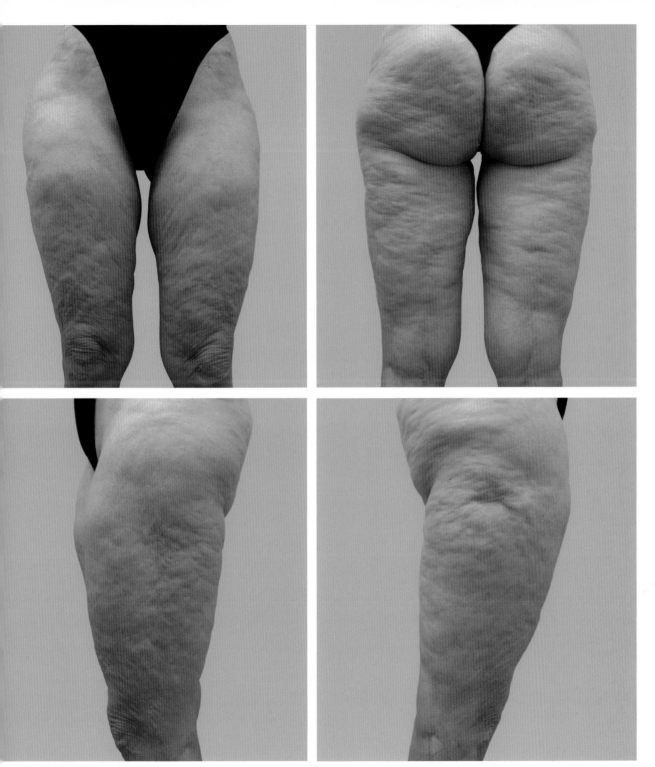

5A-5D: Woman Exhibiting Grade 3 Cellulite

Lionel Bissoon

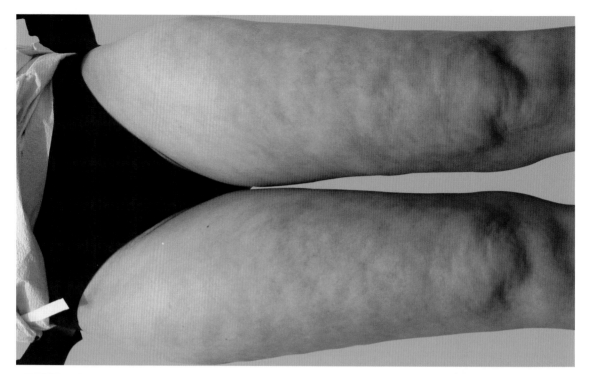

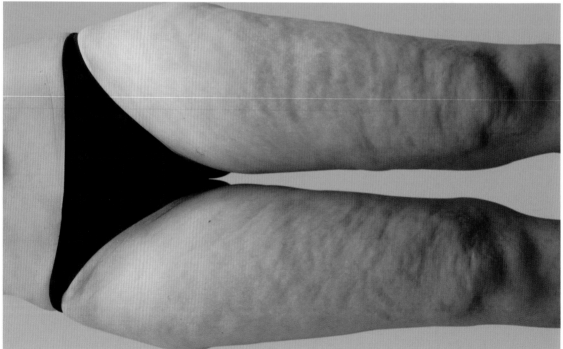

FIG. 6A-6B: These photos show a woman with severe Grade 2 Cellulite who was treated with Stringcision™, followed by three sessions of Mesotherapy.

Lionel Bissoon

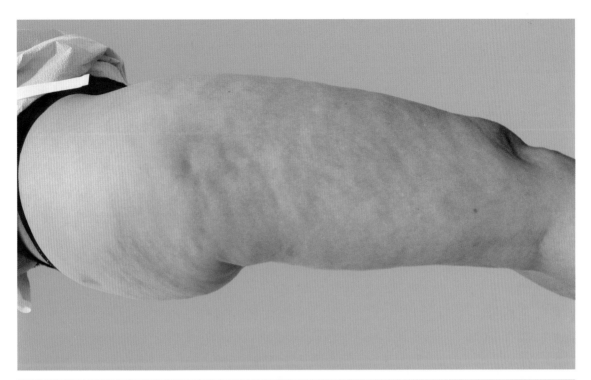

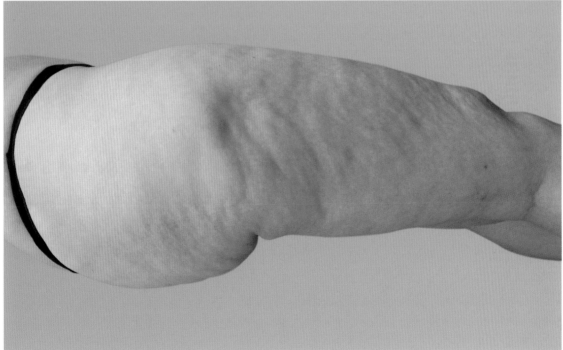

FIG. 7A-7B: This is the same woman.

Lionel Bissoon

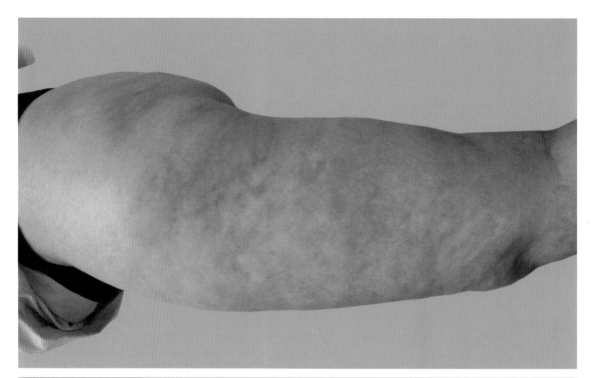

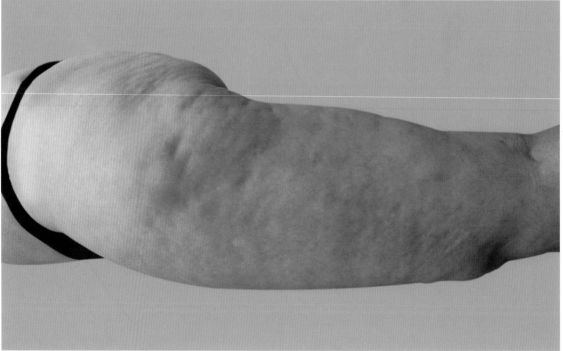

FIG. 8A-8B: This is the same woman again.

Lionel Bissoon

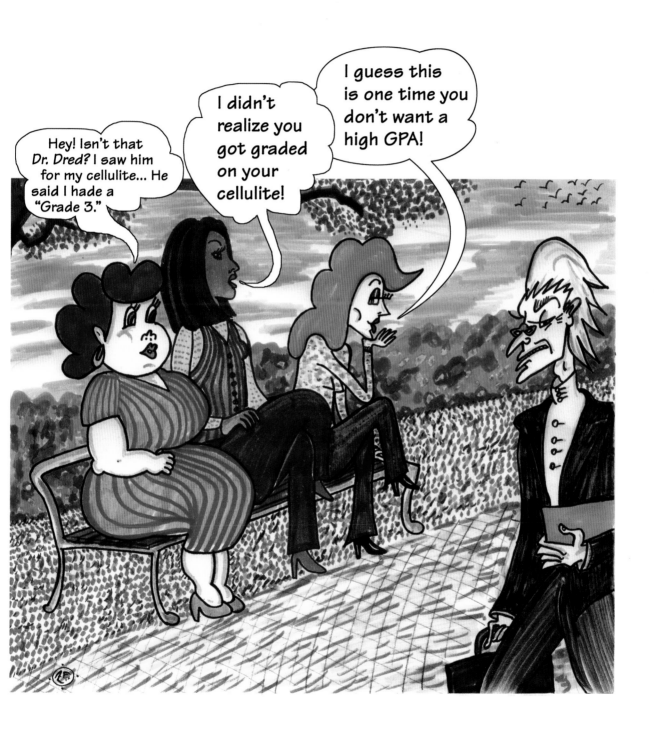

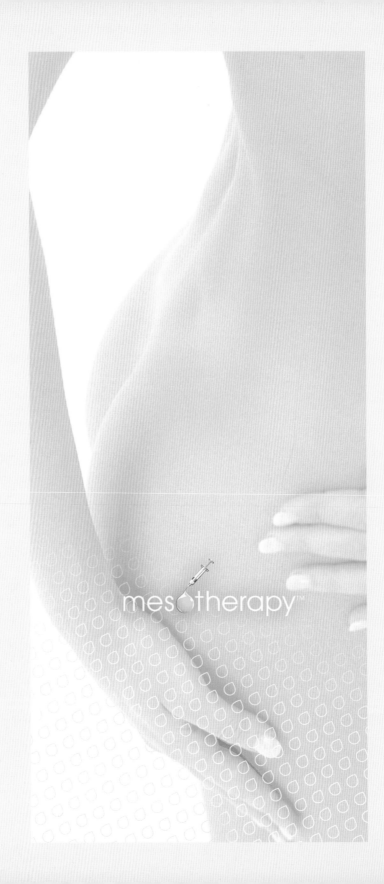

mes therapy™

5.
Mesotherapy

Mesotherapy is the practice of delivering microinjections

of conventional or homeopathic medications (and/or

vitamins) under the skin to directly treat the areas

where the condition exists. Discovered in 1952 by

Dr. Michel Pistor, it was recognized by the French

National Academy of Medicine in 1987 as an integral

part of traditional medicine. Each day, Mesotherapy is

employed by more than 15,000 doctors to treat 60,000

patients in France, and it is widely used throughout

Europe, as well as in some African and South American

countries. Mesotherapy has only recently been

introduced to the United States of America due, in large

part, to my efforts to educate and inform the public

and the medical establishment about its benefits.

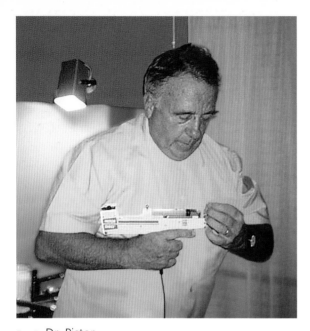

Fig. 1: Dr. Pistor
Courtesy of Dr. Petit of France

Dr. Michel Pistor summarized Mesotherapy in this way:
1. *Inject into the skin;*
2. *Inject at the site of the problem;*
3. *Inject small doses.*

"Medicinal Bullets"

"A little, not very often, in the right spot," was the mantra Dr. Pistor used to summarize the philosophy of Mesotherapy. Tiny medicinal "bullets" are delivered directly to specific targets in the body, eliminating side effects and the contraindications associated with many medications. Because the target area is reached immediately with undiluted medicine, the total amount of drugs needed is greatly reduced, and the benefits are realized more quickly.

By contrast, medication administered orally must pass through the gastrointestinal tract before reaching the bloodstream and the target organ. If, for example, a medicine is intended to treat an inflammation in the knee, only a small portion of the original drug actually arrives at the knee. A large portion of many oral or intravenously injected drugs is removed by the liver and then excreted in the urine. With Mesotherapy, a much smaller dose of the same medicine is injected with a tiny needle into the afflicted area, with the skin acting as an efficient, time-release delivery system.

When treating cellulite, multiple injections are given in rows approximately one inch apart over the affected tissues. Medications are injected into the skin because of its redundant circulation. Stated simply: the vessels of the skin loop back upon themselves, and have many microscopic pores that let substances enter and leave them. Thus, it takes approximately seven days for solutions to slowly leave the skin. With cellulite treatment, I inject at the legs—from the buttocks to the knees—delivering one drop of medication to each area. See Figure 2.

Most cellulite products or programs (creams, exercises, diets) are designed to "treat" the enlarged fat cells. This is why they fail. Targeting the damaged connective tissue is the *critical* component of an effective treatment regimen. When people claim that their products and processes can decrease the appearance of cellulite, they are referring to "fat cell shrinkage." Of course, such claims ignore the "Accordion Effect." If the user gains weight, the size of fat cells increases, and the cellulite reappears.

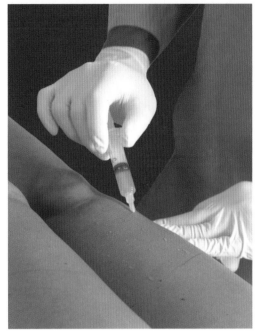

FIG. 2: This photo shows how medication is injected through Mesotherapy.

© Steven Ladner

Mesotherapy uses medications that break up damaged connective tissues, and stimulate the production of new collagen. Think of this as mending the fence. The various solutions also contain medications that help to shrink fat cells to their previous dimensions, and increase localized circulations to restore and repair damaged tissues. Basically, this is the mechanism by which Mesotherapy reduces cellulite. Hence, Mesotherapy counteracts three of the four pathological causes of cellulite— the fourth being decreased estrogen levels. See Figure 3.

TARGET: CELLULITE
Mesotherapy injections target the three out of four treatable aspects of cellulite:

- Decreased circulation

- Damaged connective tissues

- The hypertrophied (enlarged) fat cells

FIG. 3

Taking supplemental estrogen will not decrease the appearance of cellulite, nor will it restore and repair the affected areas. However, it may retard further development of cellulite. Remember, decreased estrogen leads to decreased circulation, which leads to damage to the connective tissue and fat cell herniation. You cannot replace the estrogen to treat your cellulite. I should note, however, I'm not a physician who specializes in hormone replacement. If you're considering hormone replacement, seek out an expert in this area to advise you on the pros and cons.

If you are considering hormone replacement, seek out an expert in this area to advise you on the pros and cons.

Most Mesotherapeutic formulas used to treat cellulite consist of a variety of homeopathic medications and traditional medications. All of the physicians that I have trained use the same materials in the same concentrations. Some of the medications used in

CELLULITE TREATMENT

Medications are injected one inch apart in the cellulite areas.

One drop of medication at each site will spread about one inch.

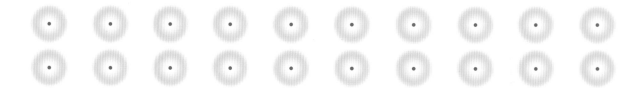

This ensures adequate distribution of medication.

Mesotherapy to treat cellulite include hyaluronidase, procaine, silica, melilotus (homeopathic sweet clover), cynara scolomus (homeopathic artichoke), aminophylline, caffeine, isoproterenol, yohimbine, vitamin C, L-carnitine, and multi-vitamins, among many others. (Some of the medications used in Europe are not available in this country, and are not FDA approved.) See Chapter 10.

I administer these medications in different combinations, and these combinations sometimes vary depending upon the doctor and the individual patient. There's nothing unusual about this. When you visit the doctor for a cold or high blood pressure, your physician has a slew of choices regarding medications to prescribe (see Chapter 10: *Mesotherapy and the FDA*, for more information). Mesotherapists also have a range of combination options from which to choose. Some physicians may have one or two treatments they prefer to use against different types of cellulite, but nearly all treatments involve some combination of the above "ingredients."

FDA Approved

Let me stress this point: The medications used in Mesotherapy are FDA-approved medications. They are being used for off-label purposes; this means that they are being used for a condition that is not listed in the label or bottle insert. Use of medications that are off-label does not violate either the spirit or letter of the law. In fact, nearly all Mesotherapy medications have well-documented safety records (see Chapter 10). The key difference between Mesotherapy and other forms of treatment is how the drugs are administered and in what amounts. With Mesotherapy, medications are injected directly into the problem areas in doses at minimal quantities that are usually much less than the FDA on-label use.

For example, if a doctor prescribed aminophylline in its oral form for someone suffering from terminal emphysema, the dose

Decreased estrogen leads to decreased circulation, which leads to damaged connective tissue and fat cell herniation.

would consist of approximately 1,000 milligrams *per day,* whereas Mesotherapy employs this same medication in dosages of approximately 100-150 milligrams *per week.* The medications used in Mesotherapy have incredible track records for safety. These same medications are used when used at higher doses for illnesses and medical conditions other than cellulite.

There are other medical conditions where medications are used for purposes other than the ones for which they were originally designed. Again, this is quite common throughout the medical world. A popular example is Botox, which is only approved for treating wrinkles between the eyebrows, but is widely used to treat crow's feet, nasal lines, neck wrinkles and a host of other conditions—including migraine headaches. Off label usage is very legal, widespread in practice and very safe in the hands of a skilled practitioner. If this was illegal every dermatologist, plastic surgeon and any physician who utilizes Botox for wrinkles and migraine headaches would be in jail.

The medications employed by Mesotherapists have been chosen because of their fundamental properties, and because of how they affect the fat cells, collagen and circulation. This use of a variety of medications to treat cellulite effectively isn't alchemy. Although individual practitioners may use proprietary drug/vitamin combinations based on what they believe is most effective in treating cellulite, all medications used are chosen because of their documented biochemical properties.

As an illustration, let's return to the drug aminophylline, which is approved for treating terminal emphysema patients. The reasons it's used for this purpose is because aminophylline exhibits alpha receptor blocking properties. By blocking the alpha receptors, it facilitates dilation of the lungs, and the patient is able to breathe. In Mesotherapy, aminophylline blocks these same alpha receptors on the fat cells, indirectly causing the breakdown of fat.

The drugs used in Mesotherapy are FDA-approved and used in smaller quantities.

(Remember, one of the causes of cellulite is increased fat cell size.) Therefore, aminophylline is a natural choice for treating cellulite. The dosage of aminophylline used in treating cellulite is quite small compared to what is administered on a daily basis for emphysema sufferers, who are very sick patients.

The Treatment Process

Here's how a typical program of Mesotherapy works, from beginning to end.

It starts when you call my office to make an appointment. When you arrive in my office, you're given a form, where you summarize your biographical information and medical history. I then perform a basic medical evaluation of your overall health status, checking your pulse, blood pressure, weight, etc. before evaluating the degree of cellulite. At this point, I grade the cellulite, looking to see if there are dimples in the buttocks and thighs—either superficial or very deep. Once this is finished, you are photographed and given an allergy test for the drug hyaluronidase. The allergy test is important because hyaluronidase is critical in helping to break up the damaged connective tissue and stimulating its repair.

Although hyaluronidase is known to produce allergies, I've seen only a handful of allergic reactions during my career as a Mesotherapist. The rash manifests as a raised wheel (rash) the size of a quarter, which is localized to the injected areas and does not spread. The size reflects the distance the medication has diffused. There is itching associated with this reaction, but topical cortisone or Benadryl relieves this itching. An oral dose of prednisone clears the rash in about two days.

I have seen 12 allergic reactions to hyaluronidase in five years. Of these 12 patients, four elected to forego further treatment. The other eight patients took prednisone (an anti-inflammatory cortisone) prior to treatment, and one or two doses post-treatment. The allergy is *rare*, but I test all patients before initiating Mesotherapy. Occasionally, a patient develops an allergy to hyaluronidase several weeks into the treatment. This is a delayed hypersensitivity reaction, which is treated with prednisone as Mesotherapy sessions continue.

After you have dressed once again, I explain how cellulite forms, and how compressive garments, exercise and diet can affect the condition. At this time I perform a panty consultation (see Chapter 8). I also discuss Mesotherapy treatment, explaining how and why the medicines are injected. The solutions are injected in rows one inch apart, each site receiving one drop of solution. Just one drop spreads out to an area approximately one inch square.

I also discuss why the injections are made into the skin. The reason: skin has what is referred to as redundant circulation, which means the circulation is essentially poor, and any medication injected into it will stay there for about seven days. By injecting medications into the skin, Mesotherapists take advantage of this "depot phenomenon."

Then, I go on to discuss pre-treatment.

I ask my patients to eat food before the session, to eat something containing protein, and I request that they do not drink caffeine before the treatment. Caffeine increases the action of the drug aminophylline (if it's used), and can make the patient feel nauseated or jittery. After we've covered pre-treatment, I discuss potential side effects.

The biggest side effect of Mesotherapy involves minor bruising *(black and blue marks)*. Nearly every patient will get black and blue marks, which will last for approximately 7-10 days following the session. Some women are shocked when told that these marks

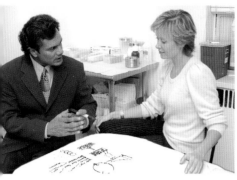
Patient Consulting with Dr. Bissoon
© Steven Ladner

will last that long. However, I point out that 7-10 days is nothing compared to suffering with cellulite for 10, 15 or 20 years. That usually puts the black and blue marks into perspective, and resolves their concerns about bruising during the 10-15 week treatment program. Some women are worried about scarring, but this simply doesn't happen.

As an example, Carol experienced minor bruising that lasted just five to 10 days following each session, as did Tina, but she described the bruising as minor. "And it cleared up quickly." Says another patient Kara, "I have very fair skin and bruise easily. I've had noticeable bruising that usually lasts about two weeks, but I haven't had as much bruising as I thought I would. Dr. Bissoon suggested that I take [a homeopathic remedy called] Arnica, which helped minimize the bruising."

Another possible side effect is skin infection. Whenever you break the skin via an injection, surgery or any form of "traumatic" procedure, there's always a chance of infection. In Mesotherapy, we follow the universal precautions of cleaning the body area with alcohol prior to treatment, as well as using gloves and disposable needles. In five years, I have never seen a Mesotherapy-related infection, and only 10 (approximately) cases have ever been reported in the medical literature during Mesotherapy's 52-year history. No serious mishaps, such as heart attack, shock or death, have ever been documented. Meanwhile, 100 people die from liposuction and related cosmetic surgery procedures each year.

(Approximately 106,000 people die from adverse drug reactions while in hospitals. Accidents claim 90,523 people per year.

The biggest side effect of Mesotherapy involves minor bruising (black and blue marks).

In the 52 year history of Mesotherapy, there have been no deaths. The question is—is Mesotherapy safe? When compared to the above statistics from 1994, it is probably the safest medical specialty in the world.)

As noted, allergies to hyaluronidase are quite rare. Any reaction is localized and benign—i.e., not life threatening. The raised rash is about the size and shape of a quarter. Aminophylline, by itself, produces no side effects. However, if the patient drinks coffee just prior to treatment, the caffeine will interact with the aminophylline, causing nausea and "the jitters" for approximately 10-15 minutes.

Post-Treatment Guidelines

Following a treatment session, the only restriction I impose is to ask women not to engage in vigorous activity for 48 hours, and to abstain from hot baths, hot tubs, Jacuzzis and massages. The reason for the abstinence is because the first 48 hours following the use of hyaluronidase is the most critical. That's when the hyaluronidase is most active, so I do restrict women from indulging in these activities. Massages, vigorous exercise and hot baths increase the circulation, and may flush the medicine immediately out of the dermis and into general circulation, dramatically diminishing the treatment's effectiveness. But those are pretty much the only post-Mesotherapy restrictions. After a session, the average patient usually goes back to work or their other normal activities.

The following restrictions apply to Mesotherapy patients for 48 hours following cellulite treatments:

✓ **No hot baths, hot tubs or Jacuzzis.**

✓ **No massages.**

✓ **No exercise or other vigorous activities.**

Birth of a Passion

My interest in Mesotherapy began five years ago, when a patient named Azar Velbinger walked into my office, and said, "Dr. Bissoon, you have to learn Mesotherapy. It will change your life."

I'd never heard of Mesotherapy, so I was skeptical. But as she explained what Mesotherapy was, and the different conditions for which it could be used, I listened intently. The next day, she came to my office, and called the French Society of Mesotherapy, asking if they would accept an American physician interested in training. Initially, they did not want to offer me the training, since I did not speak French, but eventually they acquiesced.

Earlier, I had specialized in sports medicine, but because 90% of my patients were women, many kept asking me if I could do something about their cellulite. Once I trained as a Mesotherapist, the treatment of cellulite became my obsession. After studying in Paris and London, I returned to the U.S.A. to practice Mesotherapy. Over the last four years, I returned to Paris many times in my quest to find the best cellulite treatment. Ultimately, it was left to me to champion Mesotherapy as a cellulite treatment in America, and spearhead the training of other physicians. Thanks to the growing interest in Mesotherapy, especially among women, the treatment of cellulite continues to evolve and improve lives. More importantly, I would like to thank Azar for convincing me to study Mesotherapy. Because of her persistence, thousands of women have been treated.

When I told one sports medicine patient about Mesotherapy, she became so excited, she jumped from the treatment table, and said, "Please doctor, you have to do it." Then, she literally undressed in the therapy gym, so I could examine her legs. She couldn't contain her excitement once she knew there was hope. Although she was only 27, this woman would not wear a swimsuit, shorts or a skirt.

Patients' attitudes about themselves change. I see the swift improvement in self-image and self-confidence— not to mention changes in the way they dress.

She got tremendous results after her first treatment, and by the eighth or tenth session, she was nearly cured. This dramatic result intensified my interest. I now saw hope for all the women who'd previously asked me to treat their cellulite.

Since launching my Mesotherapy practice, I have relied on word of mouth and media coverage to spread the word, and there has been no shortage of patients. Eliminating cellulite makes a major difference in women's lives, and in mine. I experience a great deal of joy treating patients, and seeing their happiness as they accomplish results over 10-15 treatments. It's truly an amazing thing to see.

Patients' attitudes about themselves change. I see the swift improvement in self-image and self-confidence—not to mention changes in the way they dress. They wear swimsuits and shorts again, without embarrassment. Friends and family are thrilled, and provide numerous compliments about their legs. Such results are very rewarding. What could be more empowering than changing somebody's state of wellness and fostering an increased sense of self-esteem? These are the kinds of things that keep me interested in Mesotherapy—a specialty that I thoroughly enjoy.

Dr. Pistor's Dream

Five years ago, I met Dr. Pistor when he made a presentation at a conference on how he had (accidentally) discovered Mesotherapy. (See Figures 1 and 5.) He did acknowledge that it was an accidental discovery, and discussed how it had progressed during the last 45 years. In a private meeting with him, he told me about his dream. "My life dream is to make Mesotherapy accepted and popular in the United States. Once this is done, I would consider my life work complete."

I remember that visit as though it occurred yesterday. I remember looking at his eyes when he said those words, and he really

"My life dream is to make Mesotherapy accepted and popular in the United States. Once this is done, I would consider my life work complete."
—Dr. Michel Pistor

believed that once his work was accepted in America, it would be accepted all over the world, giving his work much more credibility. Therefore, I made it my mission to realize his dream. Unfortunately, the good doctor died before his dream was fully realized. I was actually scheduled to meet with him, having packed press clippings and news videos highlighting the growing interest in Mesotherapy in America. I wanted to show him that his dream was unfolding—that Mesotherapy was starting to take hold in the United States. It's a shame that he never lived to realize that his desire was near completion.

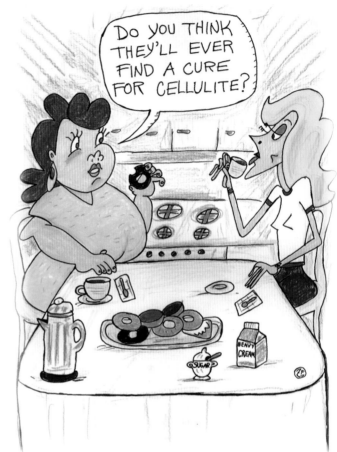

Growing Awareness vs. Mainstream Prejudice

The first physician to practice Mesotherapy in the U.S.A. was Robert Wallace, M.D. He started practicing Mesotherapy in the 1960s in New York City. See Figure 6. When I began practicing Mesotherapy, there were only two practitioners in the U.S.A., and I was one of them. Since then, as word spread in the mainstream media, people became excited, and wanted to learn more about Mesotherapy. Patients are actually taking literature to their doctors and asking them to learn this specialty, so they can be treated for cellulite. I have personally trained over 140 physicians in the last four years, and there are others traveling to Europe on a regular basis to study with the French Society of Mesotherapy. Today, there are courses appearing throughout the U.S.A., where Mesotherapy is taught on a regular basis. As awareness of Mesotherapy increases, more physicians are rushing to learn about the specialty.

Although plastic surgeons and dermatologists have no effective treatment for cellulite, some continue to criticize Mesotherapy. In a recent article questioning the validity of Mesotherapy, renowned plastic surgeon, Alan Matarasso and his colleague quote a study by a plastic surgeon in which 70% of Mesotherapy patients were satisfied with the results. A *New York Times* article on Mesotherapy and cellulite concluded, "When it comes to cellulite, hope never dies." In that same story, Vancouver dermatologist, Martin Braun said, "In my opinion it's remarkably safe, and the only thing I've seen that works for cellulite."

I must caution doctors, however, that a weekend course in Mesotherapy constitutes insufficient training—to say the least. Mesotherapy is a medical specialty designed to treat numerous conditions, and cannot be learned—much less mastered—in only two days. Unfortunately, there are unscrupulous people who are trying to fill the void by preying on unsuspecting physicians with "fast-track" courses.

Microinjection therapy, Lipoderm, Lipostabil, Lipodissolve, Needle-less Mesotherapy, and No-Needle Mesotherapy <u>are</u> <u>not</u> Mesotherapy.

Some physicians without proper (or any) Mesotherapy training are jumping on the "bandwagon," calling their programs microinjection therapy or Lipoderm. *Microinjection Therapy, Lipoderm, Lipostabil and Lipodissolve and Needle-less Mesotherapy* <u>are</u> <u>not</u> Mesotherapy. Some doctors even claim that I trained them when this simply isn't the case. If you have any doubts about your physician's credentials, call my office or visit my website at

A weekend course in Mesotherapy constitutes insufficient training— to say the least.

www.Mesotherapy.com. The site lists the doctors I have trained, at The Bissoon Institute of Mesotherapy.

Remember, not all Mesotherapists are *equally* trained. There are physicians who lead prospective patients to believe that I trained them, or tell patients they were trained by one of my associates. *I do all of my training personally!* Other physicians claim to have the most Mesotherapy experience. Thus, when someone makes a claim they have the most experience or claim to be a pioneer of Mesotherapy they are exaggerating and are not trustworthy. If your doctor makes such claims, please verify. Not all Mesotherapists are well trained. Don't choose someone just because he *claims* to be a qualified Mesotherapist.

Among the American medical establishment, there is still much ignorance and prejudice against Mesotherapy, but these prejudices—I believe—are being chipped away by a public surge of interest in Mesotherapy. Many doctors have patients who are looking toward Mesotherapy, and are demanding such treatments. In today's world, patients are educated and more interested in participating in decisions regarding their healthcare. Dermatologist and plastic surgeons have no knowledge of Mesotherapy, but some make irresponsible remarks regarding the treatment. Their attitude seems to be, "If we can't fix the problem, how can anyone else?"

Unscrupulous people are trying to fill the void by preying on unsuspecting physicians with "fast-track" courses.

What's more, since there are no other viable *Medical* cellulite treatments in this country (or anywhere else, for that matter) Mesotherapy is inspiring hope in tens of thousands of women across the U.S.A. They are asking doctors to learn the new specialty; they are asking their friends about it, and conducting research on the Internet. And, especially as major magazines and newspapers provide more information about Mesotherapy, they are learning more about it.

Not all Mesotherapists are trained equally. Don't go to someone just because he claims to be a qualified Mesotherapist. If you have any doubts, call my office or visit my website at www.Mesotherapy.com.

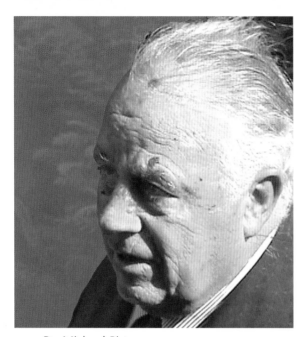

FIG. 5: Dr. Michael Pistor
Courtesy of Dr. Petit of France

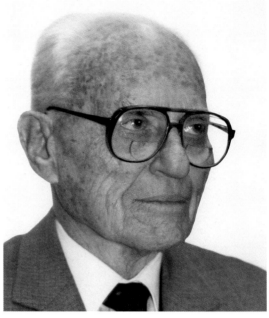

FIG. 6: Dr. Robert Wallace, the first Mesotherapy
practitioner in the U.S.A.

"I was researching cellulite on the Internet," says Carol, "and came across Mesotherapy. I desperately wanted to feel better about myself, so I took the next step."

"A Russian friend mentioned Mesotherapy, and how it is very popular in Russia," says Tina. She had done 10 treatments in Russia, and was very happy. Now, I was on a mission to find Mesotherapy here. I finally found it on the Internet, and just got lucky when I picked Doctor Bissoon."

As you can guess, the prejudices of the medical establishment are no match for the tide of women who stand to benefit. Women have lived in emotional distress, fear and shame for too many decades to allow ignorance and misconceptions to foil their hopes. After all, modern medicine in this country has done literally nothing about cellulite, so it is suffering from something of a credibility gap.

At an anti-aging conference in Chicago, my friend Ron Rothenberg, M.D., Director of Medical Education at the Bissoon Institute of Mesotherapy, pulled me aside. "I want you

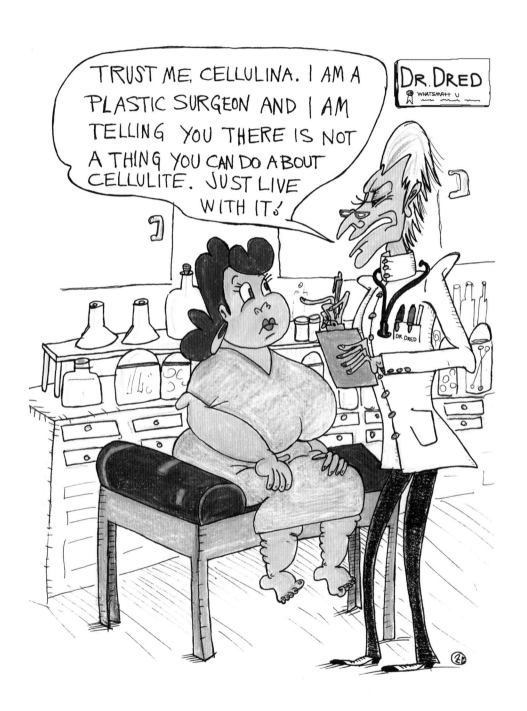

to meet Dr. Denise Bruner," he said. I thought he was joking. Dr. Bruner had been highly critical of Mesotherapy in a story published by *U.S. News & World Report*. I was somewhat surprised, therefore, when Dr. Bruner gave me a big hug, and said, "I really want to learn Mesotherapy. When can I start?" When I reminded her of the *U.S. News* article, she replied, "Honey, I did my research, and I reserve the right to change my mind with the right facts." Today, Dr. Bruner is practicing Mesotherapy in Arlington, Virginia. If the former president of the American Society of Bariatric Medicine can realize the science and benefits of Mesotherapy, then the rest will follow.

"Since Mesotherapy is not approved (by plastic surgeons in this country), they're skeptical," says Tina. "They think that if they haven't heard of it, it must be BS. With all due respect, they don't know what they are talking about. Maybe they feel this way because Mesotherapy is cheaper and takes less time. The U.S. loses out because of this skepticism toward European treatments. It's a shame because people are suffering. This treatment has been around since the '50s, so how much proof do you need that it works?"

Of course, there will always be some physicians and patients who remain skeptical about Mesotherapy, and refuse to consider the option. There are also people who continue to believe that the Sun revolves around the Earth (and the Earth is flat). The majority of those who become aware of Mesotherapy and its ability to eliminate cellulite will continue to search for treatment centers and qualified doctors. For the enlightened, it's your gain. For the ignorant and fearful, it's your loss.

Note: Many plastic surgeons around the world incorporate Mesotherapy into their practices, including some in the U.S.A.

Women have lived in emotional distress, fear and shame for too many decades to allow ignorance and misconceptions to foil their hopes.

"Since starting Mesotherapy treatments, my results have been dramatic," says Kara. "My cellulite started improving and became less apparent after my first visit. After trying every treatment out there, I initially thought I was imagining the results because I thought it was too good to be true, but after about 10 treatments I know the results are real and amazing! If you look at my before and after pictures, I don't look like the same person.

I can't begin to tell you how good I feel since I started my treatments. After spending so much money and time on every treatment out there and never seeing any results, Mesotherapy has given me the results I was always hoping for. I feel more self-confident, and no longer feel depressed when I look at my thighs in the mirror. I can actually walk in a bathing suit without the cover-up around my thighs!

It's a wonderful feeling to be able to change something in your appearance that made you feel horrible. I have taken all of Dr. Bissoon's advice. I have seen incredible results, and want to do everything I can to get the maximum benefits of Mesotherapy.

I think Mesotherapy is the most remarkable treatment out there. I wish I had known about it sooner. I would highly recommend this treatment to anyone with a severe cellulite problem like I had. This is the only treatment that has ever worked, and the results are amazing. I can honestly say that this treatment has changed my life. I have never felt better and I am absolutely thrilled to look in the mirror."

"I like what I see."

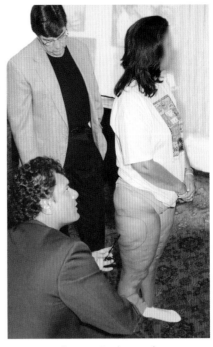

FIG. 7: Dr. Bissoon is shown here teaching plastic surgeon Tommy Guillot how to examine and grade cellulite.

© Steven Ladner

Mesotherapy • 114

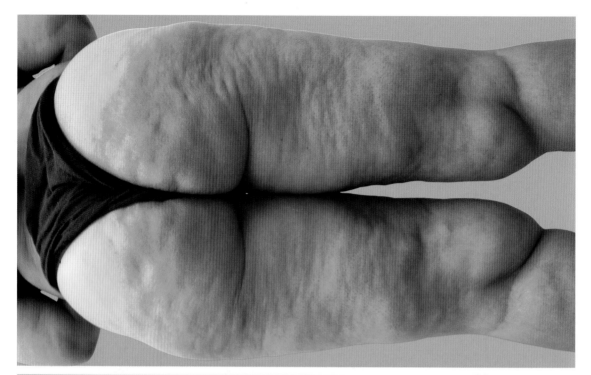

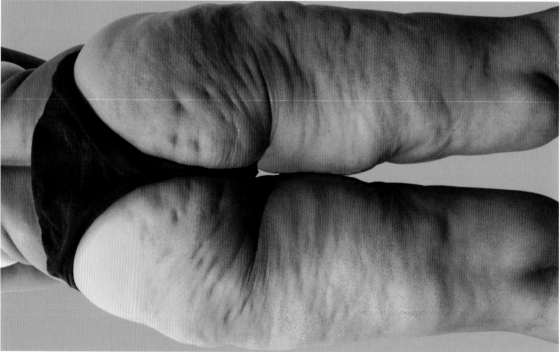

Fig. 8A-8B: This is a *back* view of a middle-aged woman had severe Grade 3 Cellulite. She was initially refused treatment. Upon patient insistence, she was treated with two sessions of Subcisions™, and two sessions of Stringcisions™ and multiple Mesotherapy sessions.

Lionel Bissoon

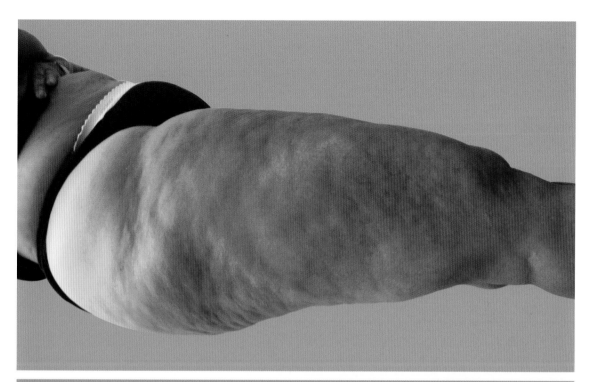

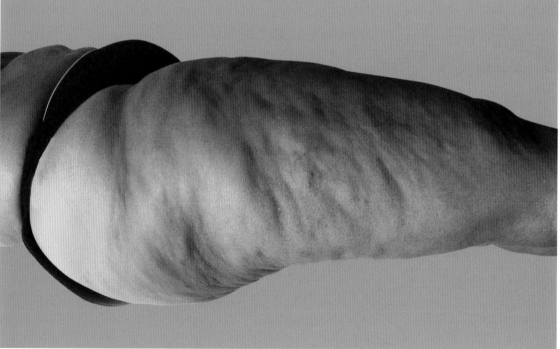

Fig. 9A-9B: The two photos show the thighs. The *before* is on the *bottom; after* is on *top.*

Lionel Bissoon

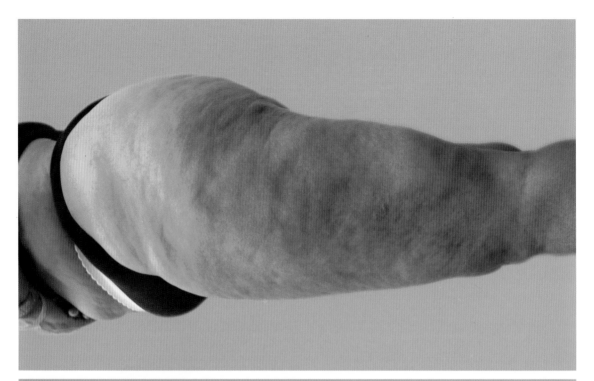

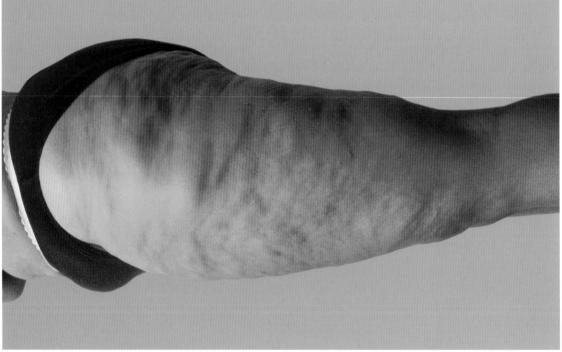

FIG. **10A-10B:** The same patient.

Lionel Bissoon

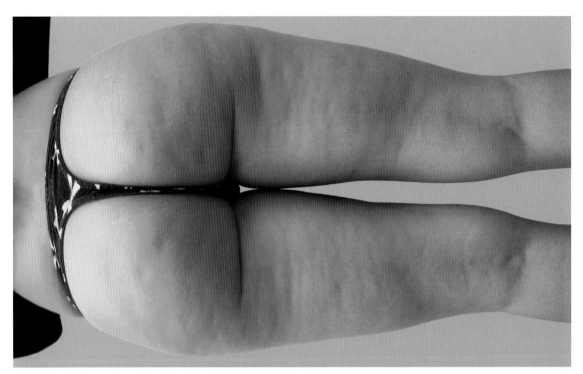

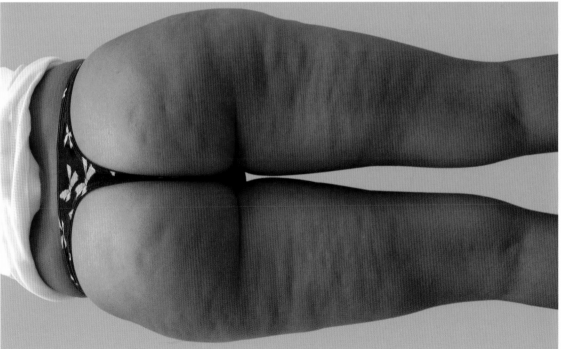

FIG. 11A-11B: This is a 28 year old woman who had 10 sessions of Mesotherapy and Subcision™ to the buttocks and saddlebags.

Lionel Bissoon

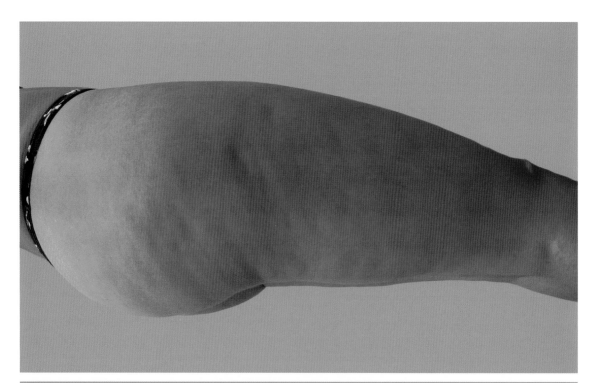

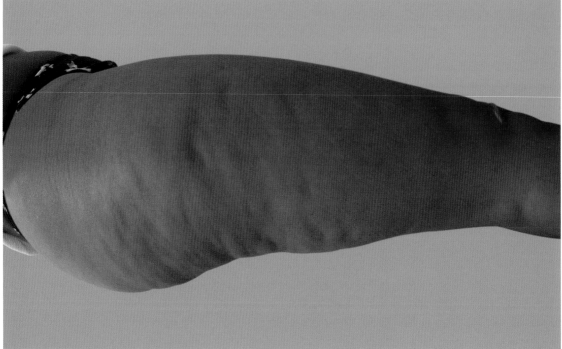

Fig. 12A-12B: This is the same patient.

Lionel Bissoon

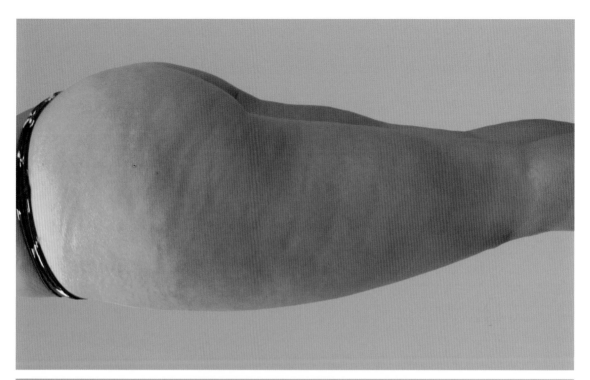

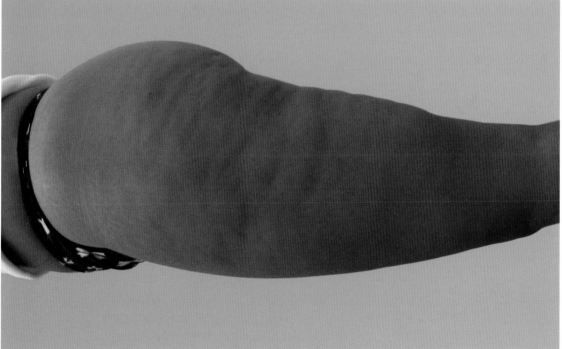

FIG. 12A-12B: This is the same woman.

Lionel Bissoon

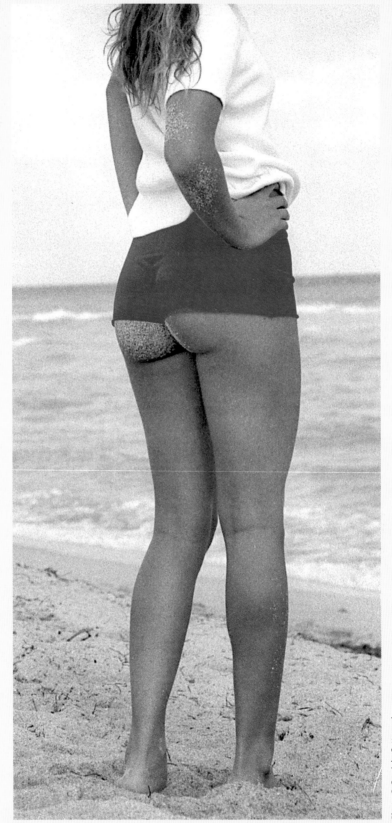

6. *All About*
Subcision™/
Stringcision™

Subcision™/Stringcision™ is another weapon in

the anti-cellulite arsenal that is combined with

Mesotherapy to treat the dimples associated with

cellulite. Like Mesotherapy, Subcision™/Stringcision™

is an outpatient procedure that targets the connective

tissues located in the subcutaneous layer, using

a special hypodermic needle. Clinical studies indicate

that the procedure is highly effective, relatively pain

free, and has a low incidence of side effects.

If dimpling is the only problem, then Subcision™/Stringcision™ is the best choice. However, if dimpling and the cottage cheese effect are both present, you will need Subcision™/Stringcision™ to treat the deep dimples and Mesotherapy to address the cottage cheese appearance. If no dimples are present, Mesotherapy is the best and only option. By itself, Mesotherapy can treat small dimples, but since large dimples require more time to treat, one or both procedures are recommended. See Figure 1.

How It Works

Before Subcision™ begins, your physician identifies the dimples he intends to treat that day, and anaesthetizes the areas with lidocaine. Next, a special needle is inserted underneath the skin, which cuts and thus releases the collagen bands that cause dimpling of the skin.

Terms such as "dimples" or "depressions" are somewhat misleading. Although your skin may appear to exhibit "depressions" in various places, the depressions actually represent the original location of your skin before the onset of cellulite—*before* fat cell herniation took place. In other words, dimples are not "sunken" skin, but skin that's remained in its proper place while the skin surrounding it has "risen" (been pushed outward).

In Subcision™, a special needle is used to puncture the skin's surface, and maneuvered under the defect to make "subcuticular" cuts or "cisions." As a result, the depression is lifted by the releasing action of the procedure, as well as stimulation of production of connective tissue that forms in the course of normal wound healing. Subcision™ produces more immediate cosmetic results than Mesotherapy alone—"instant gratification." Plastic surgeons and dermatologists recommend filling these defects with fat grafting. If only they understood that these are not genuine defects in fat deposition, but collagen fibers attaching the skin to the muscles. I must point out, the biggest setback to this procedure is black and blue marks. The discoloration usually resolves within two to six weeks in the majority of patients. Rarely does the discoloration go beyond this time frame.

I developed Mesotherapy Stringcision™ to quickly resolve unsightly dimpling in the thighs and buttocks. The procedure involves using a surgical thread (string) which is looped under the dimple and with a flossing motion the dimples are released. The procedure involves considerably less "down time" than Subcision™, though both procedures accomplish the same results. In addition, Stringcision™ produces fewer complications, a faster recovery and instantaneous results. Patients are amazed by the immediate changes in their legs. I recommend Subcision™ only for rimples, which are the shallow horizontal lines that indent the back of the legs.

Unlike Mesotherapy, which is nearly pain free, Subcision™/Stringcision™ patients may experience light to moderate pain for several days after the procedure. "With the Mesotherapy, there was some pain at first, but the swelling quickly goes away and then it's all gone." says Tina. "With Subcision™, there is a little more bruising (which also heals in a few weeks), but I didn't find it all that painful." Most patients are healed in six weeks. In rare cases, it may require three to six months for the black and blue marks to resolve.

Bruising is the most common side effect. Although most bruises begin to disappear after 10 days, 90% of patients studied reported that some bruises survived for as long as four months following Subcision™. On the plus side, almost 80% of the women studied said they were satisfied with the improvements achieved during their first session.[1] With Stringcision™, the black and blue marks begin to disappear in approximately five days. When there is

---

[1] *"Subcision: A Treatment for Cellulite," Doris Maria Hexsel, M.D., and Rosemari Mazzuco, M.D.,* International Journal of Dermatology, 2000.

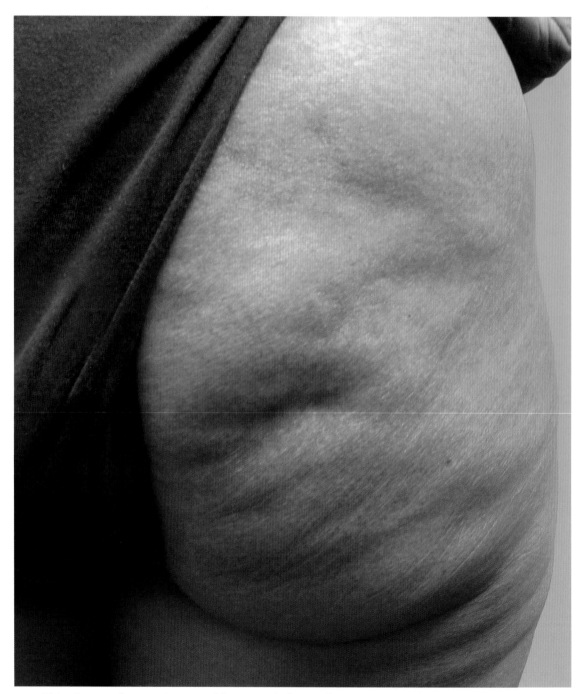

Fɪɢ. 1: This pictures shows a 35 year old woman before Subcision™. Her only concern was with the large dimple in her right buttock. This dimple could be seen through her pants.

Lionel Bissoon

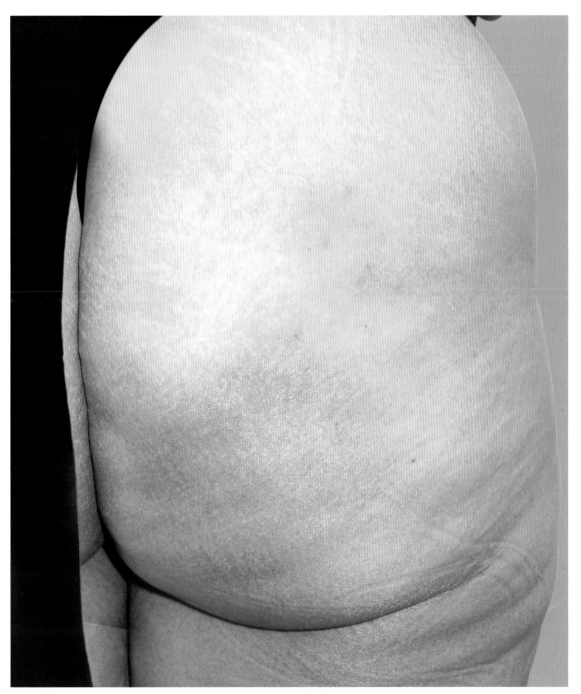

Fig. 2: This is the same patient after treatment with Subcision™.

Lionel Bissoon

prolonged bruising, a chemical peel is utilized to help resolve the bruising rapidly. In my experience, prolonged bruising is rare.

Although Mesotherapy is capable of treating the entire spectrum of cellulite, dimples require a longer treatment period. Treating deep dimples can be problematic and time consuming using traditional Mesotherapy. Because some deep dimples will not resume their original appearance with Mesotherapy alone, Subcision™/Stringcision™ is used to reduce the number of treatment sessions needed and/or to produce immediate improvement in the appearance of dimples—i.e., instant gratification. Invariably, all cellulite patients have some form of dimpling associated with cottage cheese appearance to the skin. Rarely, does one see only dimples.

If a dimple doesn't heal completely after the first Subcision™ session, another round may be necessary, but (thankfully) second sessions usually require less time and effort. Also, they are rarely needed.

As I mentioned, Mesotherapy and Subcision™/Mesotherapy Stringcision™ are sometimes combined. If a patient is exhibiting only deep dimples, I will perform Subcision™/Mesotherapy Stringcision™. However, if the patient suffers from a combination of cottage cheese appearance *and* deep dimpling, I use both procedures in tandem. I also perform Subcision™/Stringcision™ in conjunction with Mesotherapy when treating patients who exhibit deep indentations as the result of liposuction. Subcision™ and Mesotherapy Stringcision™ can be used to fix the dimpling caused by liposuction.

Despite the fact that Mesotherapy Stringcision™ is used in conjunction with Mesotherapy, Subcision™/Stringcision™ is a *surgical* procedure that requires training and skill-sets that are independent of Mesotherapy. Therefore, not all Mesotherapists are trained to perform these two procedures.

I'm not suggesting that you search for a Mesotherapist who will decide to perform one of these two procedures upon your request. Instead, you should find a physician fully capable of performing both procedures. Locating someone with expertise and experience in both modalities could be a big "plus," depending on your condition. ♦

Not all Mesotherapists are trained to perform Stringcision™.

A Letter from "Darlene"

A resident of New York City, Darlene is 40 years old, and has lived with severe cellulite for 20 years. "Dr. Bissoon told me that I had the most serious case he'd ever seen. New York is very image-conscious and body-conscious. I love to shop, but there are things I wouldn't consider wearing, because I would think, 'Just imagine what that would look like on you.' I've had a history of battling the bulges in my thighs. As they became more and more dimply, I would find ways to cover them up."

Darlene discussed her cellulite with friends, as well as different diets, but every year led to another failure. It was "'shame and more shame,' and I was tired of it." She even tried several endermologie treatments, but got no results.

One evening, she watched an episode of ABC's *20/20*. "It concluded that Mesotherapy 'might make a difference.' That was what I heard the loudest."

Since undergoing Mesotherapy, Darlene has been amazed at the smoothness of her legs, comparing her before-and-after appearance to night and day. "It's been a long process . . . but when I look at my legs, I see a difference. It's a feeling of, 'Yes! One dream is going to come true.' It's getting closer to reality. I can go in a store, and pick out things that I can wear above the knee."

"Would I recommend Mesotherapy to others? **Yes,** I absolutely would! I would say to people, you will **see** the difference."

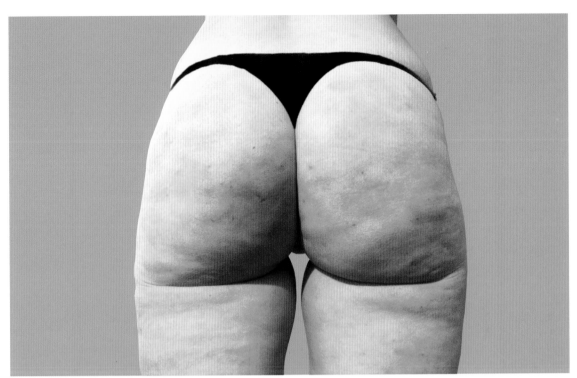

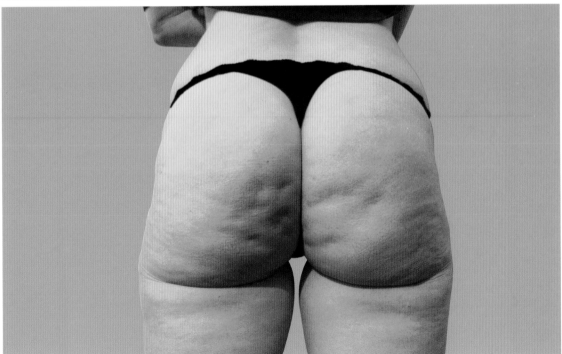

FIG. 3A-3B: This woman underwent Liposuction but still had dimples, post-Liposuction. She was treated with Stringcision™. Picture A *(bottom)* is *before;* Picture B *(top)* shows results two weeks later. You can still see some residual black and blue in the photo.

Lionel Bissoon

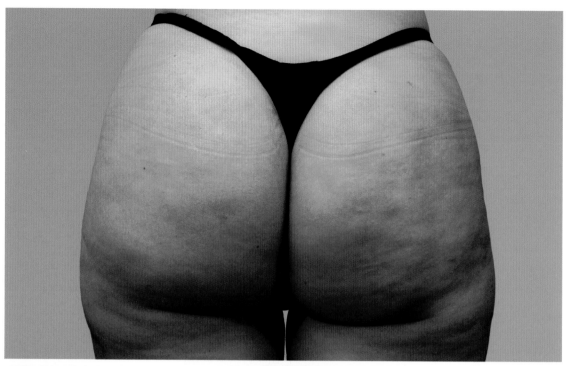

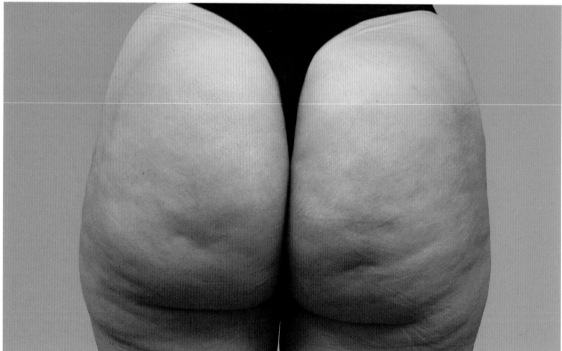

FIG. 4A-4B: This woman's dimples were treated with Stringcision. Figure A *(bottom)* is the *before,* Figure B is *after.*

Lionel Bissoon

131 • **Subcision™/Stringcision™**

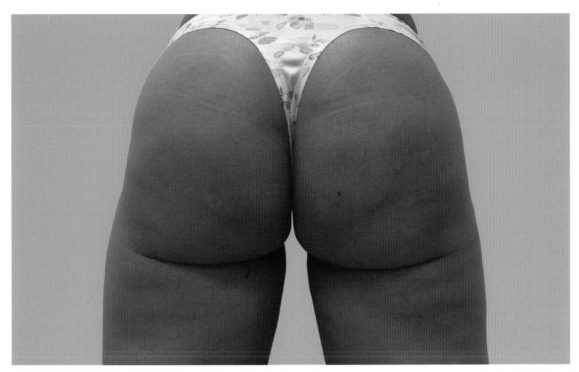

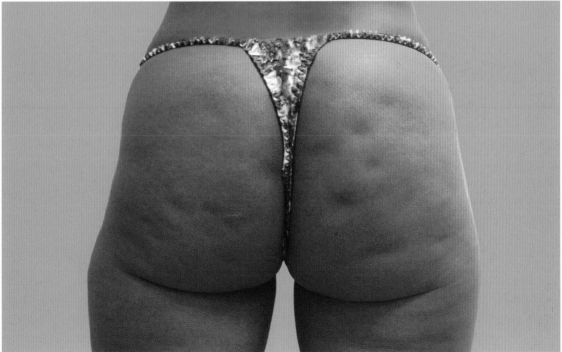

Fig. 5A-5B: This patient initially came for Mesotherapy, and did not want a full course of treatment. She then had Liposuction; several weeks later had Subcision™ to fix the dimples in her buttocks. (The *bottom* photo is the *before*.)

Lionel Bissoon

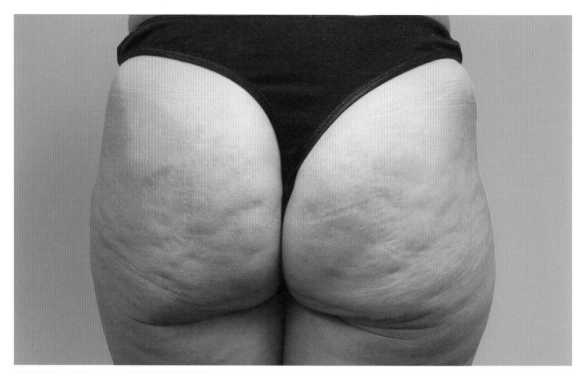

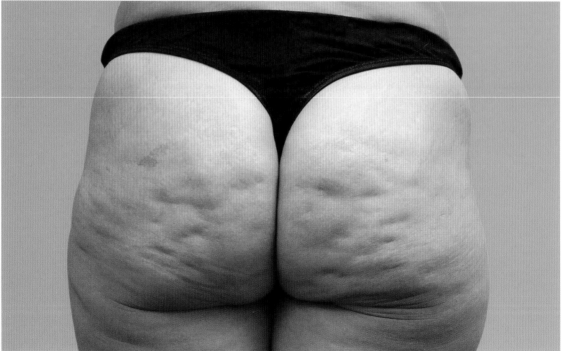

Fig. 6A-6B: This woman's dimples were treated with Stringcision. (The *bottom* photo is the *before*.) The *top* photo is after.

Lionel Bissoon

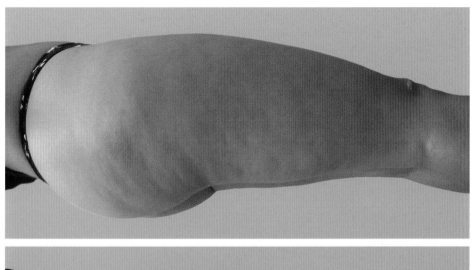

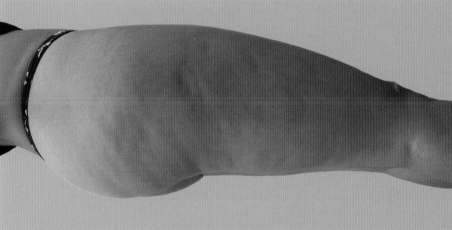

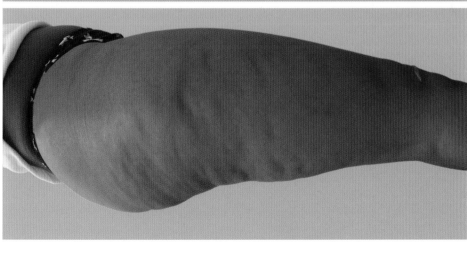

FIG. 7A-7C: This series offers a comparison view showing Mesotherapy treatment results combined with Subcision™/Stringcision™. Picture A (*bottom/left*) is her facing left *before*. Picture B (*middle*) shows the patient after 10 sessions of Mesotherapy. For Picture C (*right/top*), Subcision™ was used to fix the deep dimple in the saddlebag.

Lionel Bissoon

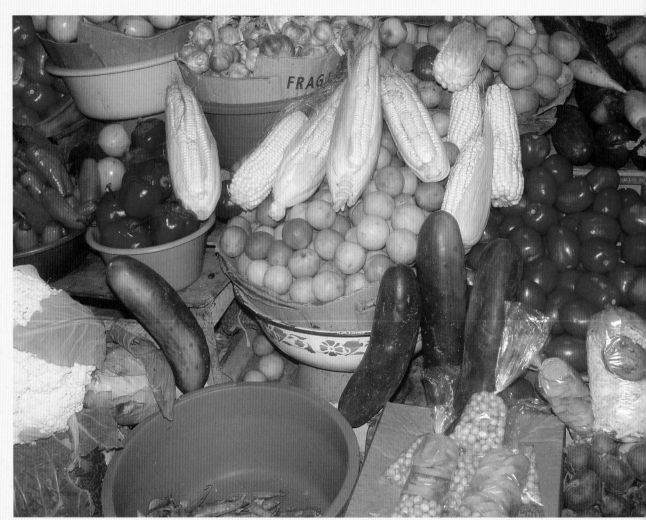

Lionel Bissoon

7. *Cellulite Prevention:*
Diet

There is little evidence that a healthier diet can actually cure cellulite once it has appeared. However, I'm not saying that a healthy diet won't prevent cellulite from forming, or keep it at bay following Mesotherapy. On the contrary, there's every reason to believe that the "domino effect of damage" is partially triggered by poor dietary habits. In fact, one of the chief culprits behind cellulite may be the justly maligned Standard American Diet—or S.A.D. Dermatologists, plastic surgeons, the media and other "cellulite gurus" insist on diet and exercise, but don't understand the nature of cellulite. The blind are leading the blind.

Yes, decreasing estrogen levels lead to malfunctioning micro-circulation, which initiates the whole degenerative process that culminates in fat cell herniation. But what causes estrogen levels to drop, and why do fewer women in the developing world suffer from cellulite? It's likely that women living in "primitive" agricultural communities are less prone to cellulite because they eat large quantities of organic foods, comprising of plant materials with estrogen-like chemicals. It is a known fact that estrogen starts to decline around the ages of 25-35. This data, obtained from studies on osteoporosis, indicates that the decline of estrogen is a slow process that speeds up as a woman approaches menopause.

It's ironic that the United States spends more money on cancer research than any other country, but that people in some of the world's poorest nations experience lower rates of certain diseases—simply because they can't afford to eat as "well" as Americans. Doesn't it strike you as odd that a "poor man's diet" could prove a better tool for prevention of disease than the medical treatments we've developed at a cost of billions of dollars?

It really shouldn't be surprising. After all, you are what you eat. Or, to use a phrase favored by computer programmers: "garbage in; garbage out."

The Alpha and Beta of Weight Gain

Most Americans don't know the Standard American Diet is called the "S.A.D." diet, but it's a truly sad diet. You couldn't invent a diet that could do a better job of promoting obesity and myriad health problems than the one most Americans eat every day. The Standard American Diet is high in processed foods, sugar and unhealthy fats, and is low in complex (plant) carbohydrates and fiber. When you eat S.A.D., you're on a fast track to weight gain—especially if you are female.

(Several years ago, I attended a conference where the former head of nutrition at the National Institute of Health called the American stool the most expensive. I was shocked, but then decided that he was kidding. However, he went on to explain that we Americans consume large quantities of vitamins and minerals in pill form, most of which are not absorbed, but excreted in the feces. He also described how deficient our foods are in various nutrients.)

Remember, research has demonstrated that in most women, fat cells in the buttocks, thighs and knees have a greater proportion of fat-storing alpha-2 receptors, and a smaller percentage of fat-releasing beta receptors, than the fat cells located elsewhere in the body. From the waist down, women have a ratio of one beta receptor for every seven alpha receptors. See Figure 1.

Men have a 1-to-1 ratio of alpha-receptors to beta-receptors (lucky bastards), with the exception of a newly discovered alpha-2 receptor located around—you guessed it—the stomach and intestines. Hence, women are genetically predisposed to the pear shape while men display the famous potbelly.

S.A.D.

The correlation between weight gain and cellulite is indirect, there is more of a correlation with the formation of cellulite and the SAD diet. Our ability to quickly gain weight, the preponderance of artificial chemicals and toxins in our foods, and the inability of our bodies to effectively remove those chemicals and toxins, are directly related to the Standard American Diet. Garbage in: garbage out.

One hundred years ago, the American diet was far different than today's. At that time, your general store contained very little processed food. Instead, the shelves were largely stocked with organic vegetables and fruits, seeds and grains, along with food that was canned and boxed. At the beginning of the 20TH century,

Most Americans don't know that the Standard American Diet is called the "S.A.D." diet.

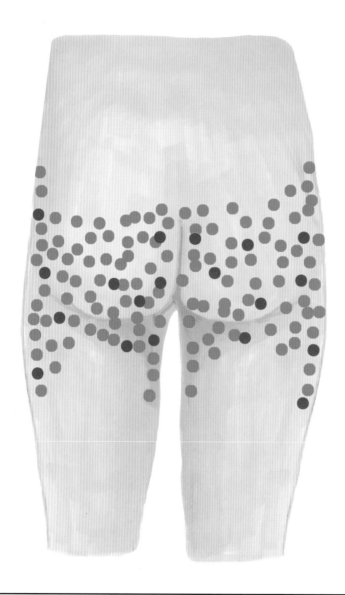

Ratio of Beta to Alpha Receptors:

● Beta Receptors   ● Alpha Receptors

Fɪɢ. 1: The Alpha-to-Beta receptors ratio in a woman's body is
approximately 7:1.

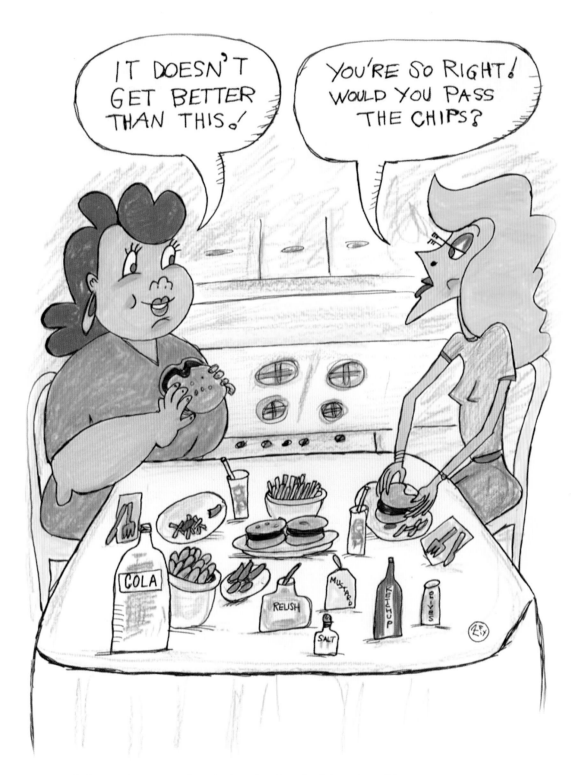

Fig. 2: Cellulina and Anna Rexia Enjoying the Standard American Diet

people grew food in their gardens or on their farms. Aside from the wealthiest citizens, people ate less meat than today, and what they did eat did not have hormones injected into it. In addition, the breads, cakes and cookies of the era did not contain partially hydrogenated vegetable oils, tropical oils and high-fructose corn syrup—staple ingredients in contemporary processed, fast foods and junk foods.

As just one example of how our bodies deal with a relatively new ingredient, let's take a quick look at high-fructose corn syrup (HFCS). HFCS is six times sweeter than sugar, helps prevent frozen foods from developing freezer burn, and keeps packaged foods soft and fresh tasting for longer periods. In the 1970s, it began making its way into foods that used to be made with sugar or contained no sweeteners at all. (Those of you who remember the 1970s will recall that the price of sugar skyrocketed.)

Today, HFCS comprises 9% of the average adult's energy intake.

According to journalist Greg Critser, author of the book *Fat Land,* the body metabolizes concentrated fructose differently from sugar, more easily converting it into fat. In fact, science isn't quite certain how the body metabolizes HFCS, but it does seem to raise levels of triglycerides, which contribute to the advent of heart disease. Also, any high-sugar diet may overload our sensitive sugar-control mechanisms, draining our systems of essential trace minerals that help maintain stable blood sugar levels, thus straining our ability to create insulin. It's probably no coincidence that the rapid spread of diabetes has occurred simultaneously with the growth of HFCS in processed foods.

Other artificial food products—including colorings, flavorings, preservatives and pesticides—may confound or overload the body's system for digesting and detoxifying foods. Over the generations, our bodies have developed enzymes that are aided by the antioxidants contained in various vitamins and minerals. These enzyme mechanisms have evolved as our diets have evolved—slowly. In just the last generation, however, the food industry has introduced thousands of new additives that have outstripped the ability of these enzymes to digest and detoxify.

As a result, we are witnessing increased tissue damage and fluid retention, caused by the blocking action of the enzyme system and a build-up of artificial food products in the body. The Standard American Diet lets us gain weight quickly and retain fluids, which negatively affect veins, lymph vessels and microcirculation—setting the stage for the formation of cellulite.

Anti-Cellulite Diets?

Although some physicians beg to differ, I don't believe there is a true anti-cellulite diet. I do believe that it's important that people have a sensible diet. And it is important that you become knowledgeable about what you eat, and how your diet effects changes in your body. But diet alone will not do the trick— not for cellulite.

For my patients, I recommend a high-protein diet that is low-to-moderate in carbohydrates and fat. However, this diet isn't going to make an appreciable difference once cellulite has appeared— though it may, indeed, retard its progress. As a general rule, I also recommend that you increase the percentage of whole foods in your diet. When possible, eat uncooked, unprocessed fruits and vegetables. In other words, eat an organically grown apple instead of applesauce. Whole fruits and vegetables contain more vitamins and other nutrients than cooked ones, and they are higher in fiber.

While you're at it, don't forget that the women in those rural South American towns are eating significant quantities of yam, yucca and soy—plants that contain phyto-estrogens. I don't believe that any cellulite diet would work unless it involved

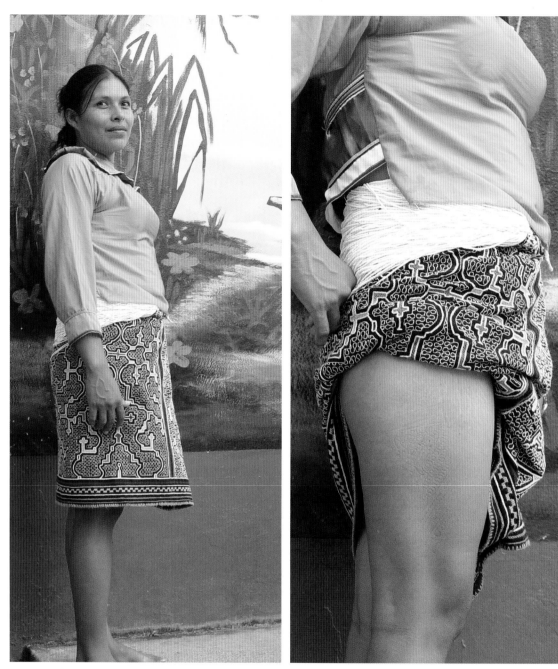

FIG. 3A-3B: The *top* photos of a Shipibo woman in her late 20s, mother of two with no cellulite. These photos of Shipibo women in Peru demonstrate the importance of a diet rich in organic foods. Additionally, these women are not sedentary in their everyday lives. Modern technology plays a little-to-no part in their activities of daily living. In contrast, their American counterparts depend heavily on modern technology for all aspects of daily living—thus becoming more sedentary with their lifestyles. The Standard American Diet is based on processed foods with multiple additives.

Lionel Bissoon

eating like an Amazonian. Dr. Barry Sears' Zone Diet and Oz Garcia's Paleolithic Diet are the only two diets which closely resemble the diets of the Amazonian people.

My recommended diet is not a cellulite-prevention diet; it's a prescription for sensible eating. I don't believe that any cellulite diet would work unless it involved eating like an Amazonian.

Eating healthier is hardly radical advice. It certainly can't hurt, and certainly can improve your overall health and appearance. There are people who have touted anti-cellulite diets in the past, and others who continue to do so. If these diets worked, millions of women would not still be suffering from cellulite. ◊

Cellulite Prevention

General recommendations to help with prevention of cellulite:

1. Decrease the amount of sugar and refined sugar in your diet.
2. Increase your consumption of leafy green vegetables.
3. Increase your consumption of fish as a source of protein.
4. Consume as many cruciferous vegetables as possible.
5. Eat a diet high in soy content.
6. Eat as much organic foods as possible.
7. Decrease your consumption of red meat.
8. Exercise 20-25 minutes every other day.
9. Take the stairs instead of using elevators.
10. Whenever possible, walk instead of driving.

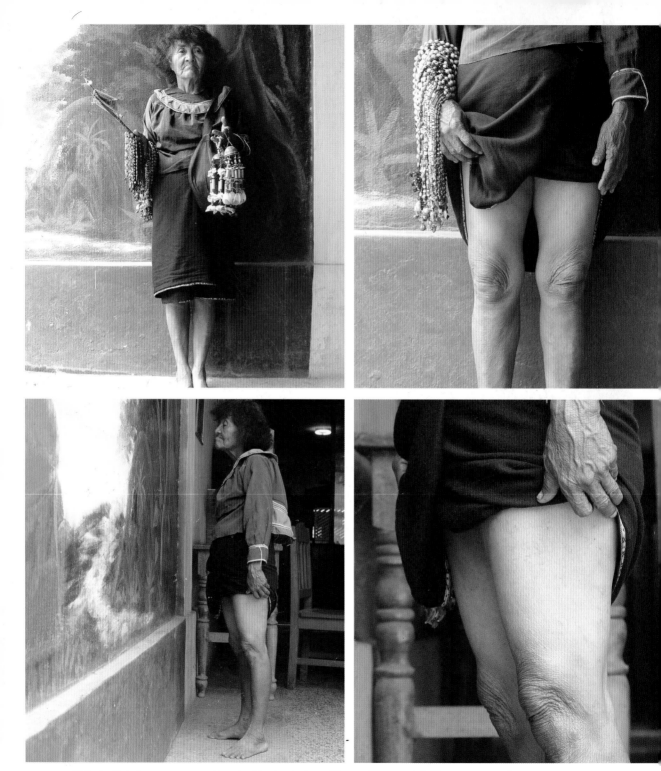

FIG. 4A-4D: Elderly Shipibo woman estimated to be in her 60s—with no cellulite.

Lionel Bissoon

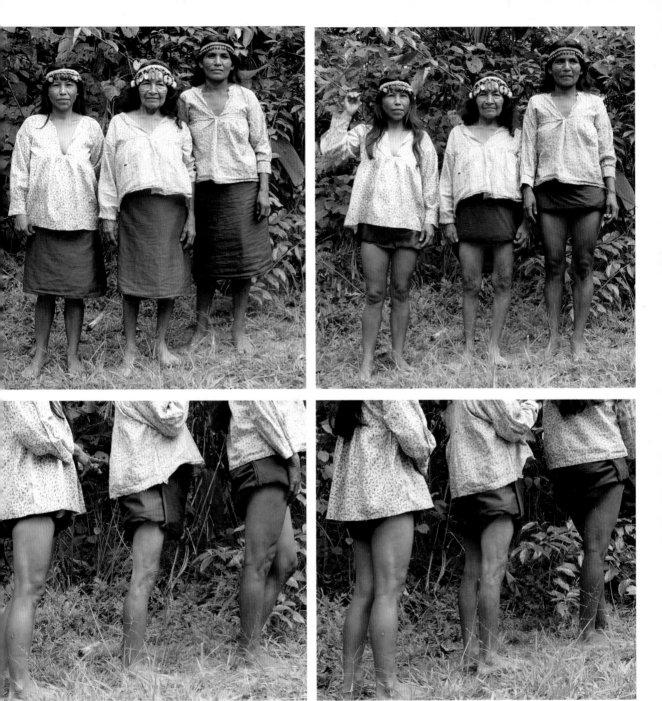

5A-5D: Jaibro women in the Amazon without cellulite. The woman on the *left* is 38 years old, the *middle* one is 57 and the one on the *right* is 35.

Lionel Bissoon

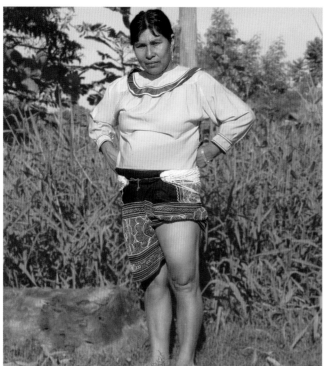
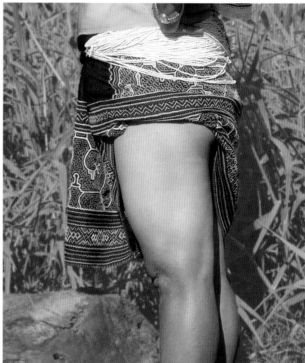
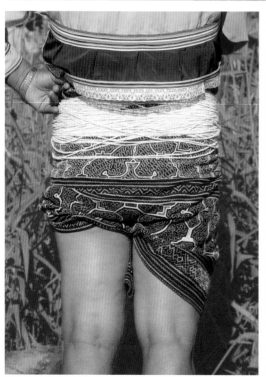
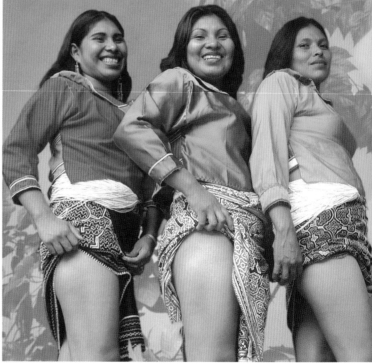

FIG. 6A-6D: First three photos show a middle-aged Shipibo woman, mother of four, no cellulite. On the *bottom right* three daughters of the first woman—no cellulite.

Lionel Bissoon

147 • Cellulite Prevention: Diet

A Letter from "Stephanie"

At 29, Stephanie lives in Davie, Florida, where she enjoys working out, eating out, attending sporting events, movies and the theater.

"I first noticed my cellulite when I was in high school. It was on my outer thighs. I think it got worse—just more dimples in that area. I also had dimples on the backs of my legs, so I rarely wore very short shorts, and if I did, I was very cognizant of how my legs looked. There was one huge dimple, which I called 'the crater,' on my right leg. I always tried to hide that one.

"I had a very normal love life growing up. I had relationships and boyfriends—it was all normal. But when it came time for sexual intercourse, I always walked around a certain way when I was naked to make sure my cellulite could not be seen—whether it was 'having an itch' on the back of my leg to cover the cellulite . . . or grabbing a blanket because I was cold (when I wasn't)! Looking at the front of my naked body, I looked great. From the back, I hated it.

"When I met Dr. Bissoon, I told him I had the most severe cellulite in the world. He said he would give me an award if I did. He examined me, said there was good news and bad news. The good news: cellulite was totally treatable. The bad news: I didn't win the award.

"Of course, anybody who's had cellulite has their array of cellulite creams, lotions and oils in their bathroom. I even tried taking these specific vitamins, which my health magazine recommended to cure cellulite. I tried cellulite cream with a loofah to scrub those dimples away. I bought a massager to massage the dimples away. I had a consultation for endermologie, and almost did that, but it's not permanent.

What kinds of results did earlier treatments provide? ***"No results!!"***

A Letter from "Stephanie" (Continued)

"When I went for the endermologie consult, the lady recommended a Mesotherapy session—one injection into that 'crater' on the right leg. I left, and went directly on the Internet to research Mesotherapy. I found Dr. Bissoon, and read that he was the one who brought Mesotherapy to the States—that he was the 'teacher' of this procedure. I scheduled my consultation, and drove 90 minutes to see him.

"Yes, I had bruising from Mesotherapy; everyone does. I did have Stringcision™ on a couple of the dimples, and that left discoloration on the legs for about six months. I was upset, but Dr. Bissoon and his staff assured me it would go away, and even sent me some topical treatments that worked wonders.

"***The crater is gone!*** All my cellulite is gone! I still can't believe it. I can wear short skirts or shorts with no worry that cellulite is showing. When I walk around naked, I don't feel insecure. Especially in a bathing suit, I feel wonderful. I now walk to the steps of a pool, and get into it like a 'normal person.' I used to dive into the deep end, so I didn't have to walk around the pool.

"I've also adopted some of his recommendations on underwear. I no longer wear underwear at night, and I'll wear a G-string with a skirt or something, but I rarely even wear underwear now."

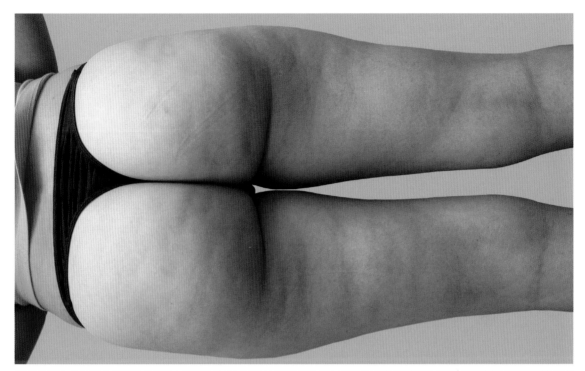

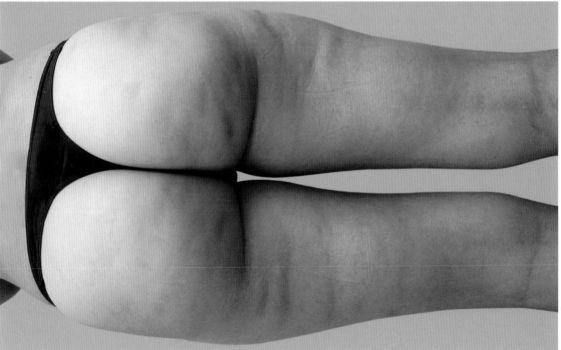

FIG. 7A-7B: This photo shows a 28 year old woman with cellulite. The patient was embarrassed to wear swimsuits. She tried extensive diet and exercise programs without success. She was treated with Mesotherapy and Stringcision™. She uses the Mesolysis™ Cellulite cream for maintenance.

Lionel Bissoon

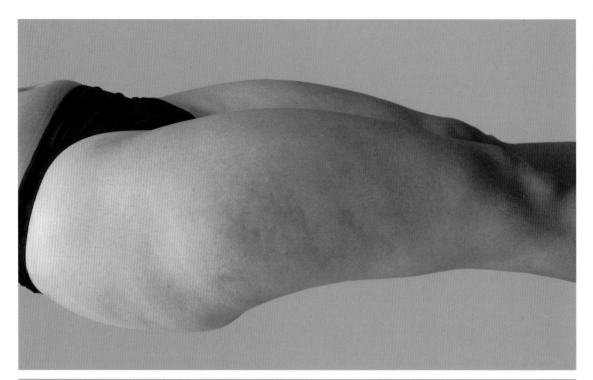
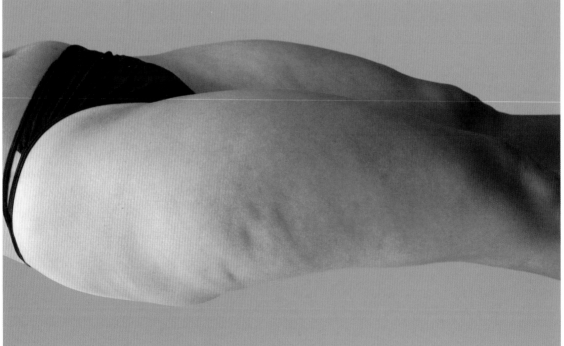

FIG. 8A-8B: This three-quarters view shows the same woman.

Lionel Bissoon

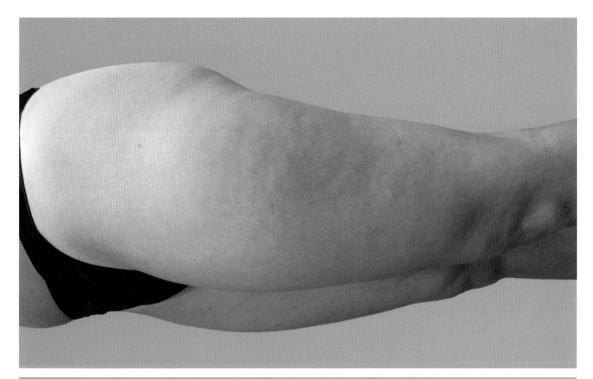

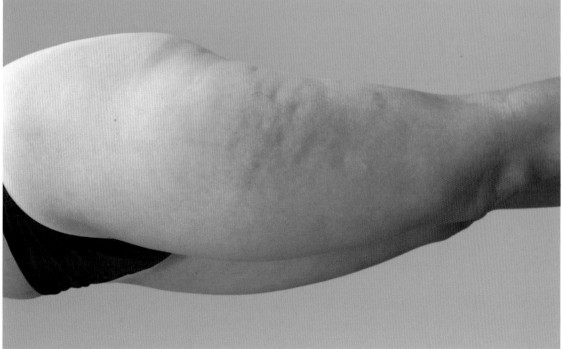

FIG. 9A-9B: This photo shows the same woman.

Lionel Bissoon

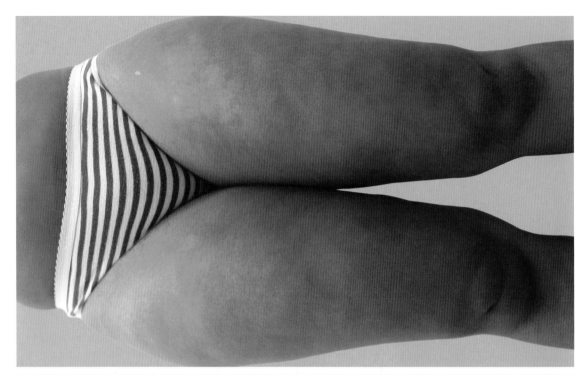

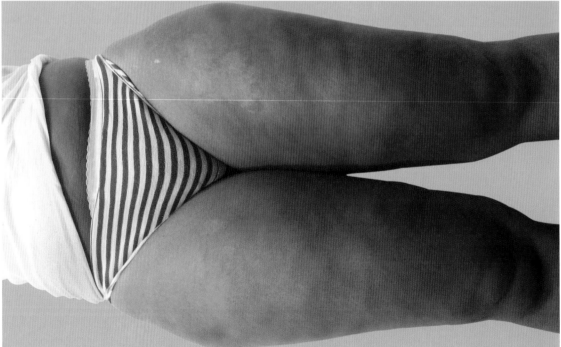

FIG. 10A-10B: This photos shows a 25 year old woman who was treated with 13 sessions of Mesotherapy by another physician—with no results. I treated her with 14 sessions of Mesotherapy. The last seven sessions were largely focused on her reducing saddlebags.

Lionel Bissoon

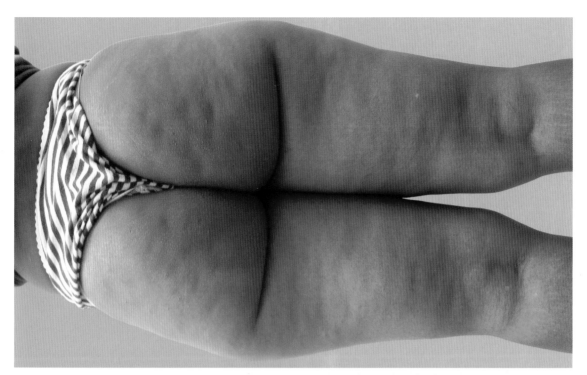

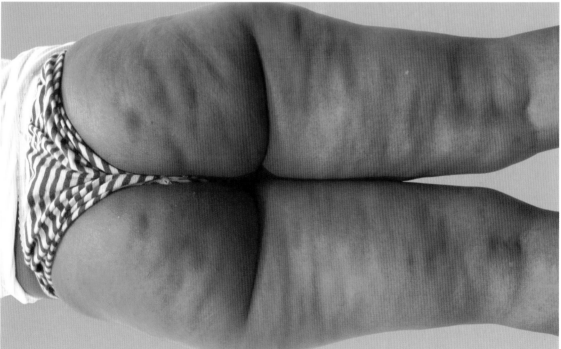

Fig. 11a-11b: The *bottom* photo shows a *back* side view of the same patient, *before*. The *top* photo shows the results *after*. The residual dimples were subcised. (That photo not yet available. Please see second edition of book in due out in 2008.)

Lionel Bissoon

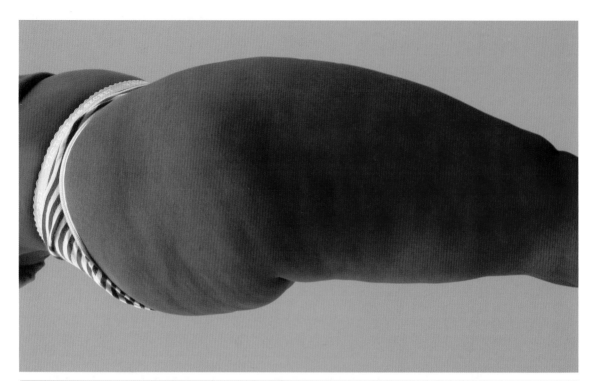

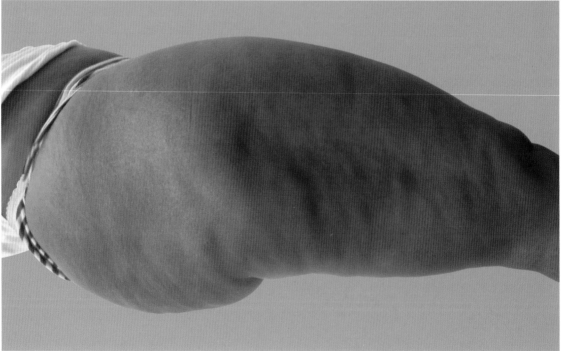

Fig. 12A-12B: The *bottom* photo is patient's *before*. *Top* photo shows the results *after*.
Lionel Bissoon

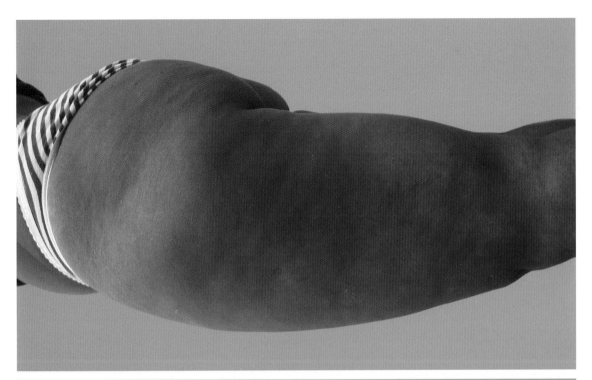

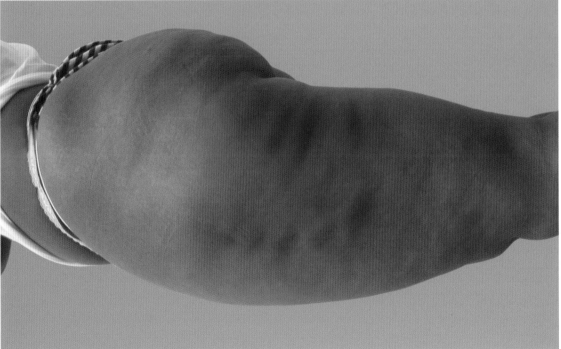

FIG. 13A-13B: The *bottom* photo shows the before. *Top* photo shows the results *after*.

Lionel Bissoon

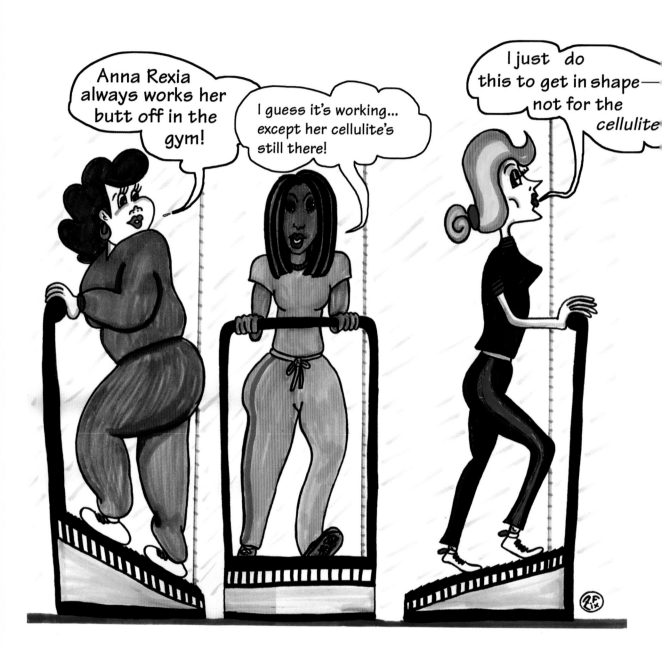

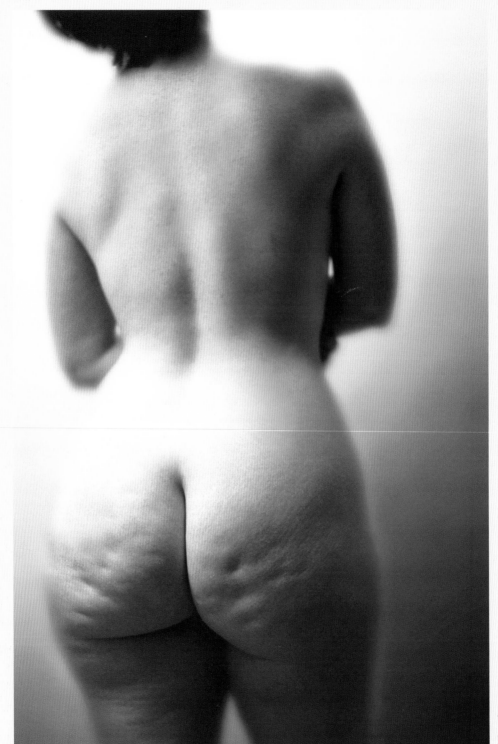

8. *The Problem with* Panties

Body chemistry aside, the biggest (and preventable) malefactor in cellulite formation is the wearing of tight undergarments. One of the few reasons I would refuse treatment to a cellulite patient is if she insisted on wearing underwear that continues to damage and/or exacerbate her condition. Why should I be expected to douse the fire when the patient is pouring gasoline on the flames?

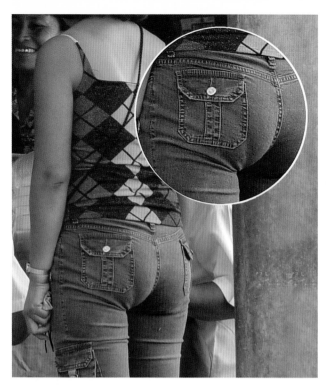

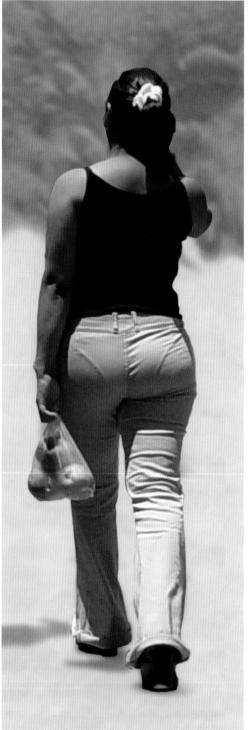

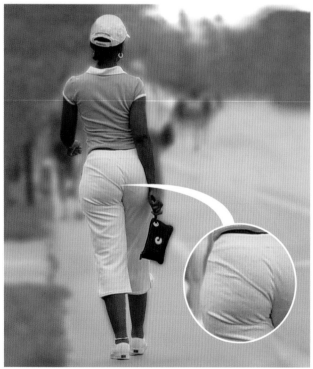

FIG. 1A-1C: Note visually obvious panty lines.

Lionel Bissoon

161 • The Problem with Panties

Most women begin wearing what I call "traditional" or "grandma underwear" as young girls. This underwear contains elastic that stretches taut across the buttocks and upper thighs, constricts the flow of blood and compresses the lymphatic vessels. In other words, the underwear itself helps to launch "Mission Cellulite."

Although such underwear is extremely damaging, many patients have no idea that it contributes to cellulite formation. It rarely occurs to them that their dimples are more pronounced on the buttocks and beneath the panty lines because of the compression caused by their underwear. In nearly five years of treating cellulite, I've noticed that women who wear "regular" underwear have more dimpling in the area of the panty lines. The longer they wear this type of underwear, the deeper the dimples become, and the more difficult they become to treat. See Figure 1.

Hardly a day goes by when I don't see a woman with visible panty lines strolling down the street. I often feel like tapping her on the shoulder, and explaining how those panty lines contribute to the development of quilted thighs and cottage cheese buttocks. Obviously, I'm not stupid enough to get arrested for what would be construed as sexual harassment. (Does the Good Samaritan Act apply to free medical advice?) Still, it would be nice if I could offer a friendly, non-threatening warning to those female passersby. The effort might save a few women from developing cellulite.

Cellulite CSI

Some women believe that tight underwear provides more support in the buttocks. This may be so. Tighter underwear may offer a little lift, but when I see panty lines peeking through clothing, I can only imagine the severity of the compression across the wearer's lymphatic tissues. Think of those microscopic vessels as a hose. The hose is turned on, and is efficiently draining

It rarely occurs to them that their dimples are more pronounced on the buttocks and beneath the panty lines because of the compression caused by their underwear.

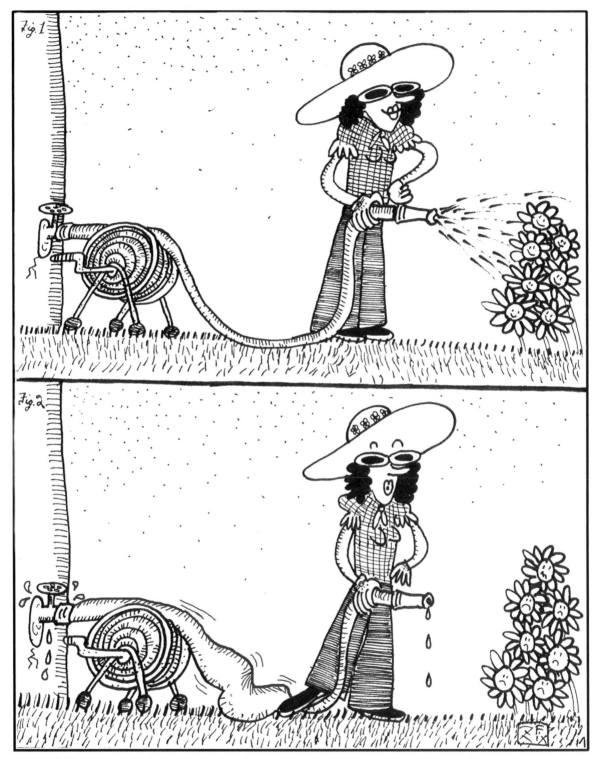

Fig. 2: This illustration depicts the severity of compression across the buttocks from the elastic panty lines.

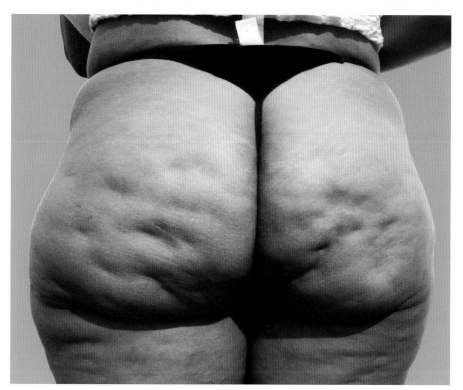

Fig. 3: Photo of a patient who has worn underwear with elastic across the buttocks her entire life. One can actually see the dimples oriented to the contour of the panty lines.

Lionel Bissoon

toxins from the various cells. Suddenly, someone pinches the hose. The water backs up, and before long it's leaking through the faucet. This is what happens when you wear tight underwear. See Figure 2.

You are compressing the tissues of your buttocks and thighs 24 hours a day, seven days a week. Eventually, this compression "works its magic," and is made manifest as dimples. Based on the depth and severity of dimpling, I can tell you approximately how long you've worn these types of compressive garments. (It's similar to the deductive analysis used by crime scene investigators, who determine a victim's time of death by studying insect activity, liver temperature, etc.)

Tight undergarments are the friends of cellulite. Choose your friends carefully: do not wear this kind of underwear.

Women are shocked when I explain the significance of wearing compressive underwear. More than once, I've threatened to stop Mesotherapy treatment for women who have refused to make the shift to cellulite-friendly underwear. The best advice I can give to any woman with cellulite, or worried about cellulite, is this: "*Please!* Stop wearing compressive underwear that produces panty lines. Not only are panty lines cosmetically unappealing, they are physically dangerous with regard to cellulite development."

Tight undergarments are the friends of cellulite.

Choose your friends carefully: do not wear this kind of underwear.

Not only do panty lines fuel dimple formation, wearing this kind of underwear while walking is even more dangerous. The movements that comprise walking can be divided into two stages of gait. The *swing* stage accounts for 40% of the gait cycle, while the *stance stage* comprises 60%. During the swing stage, the hip moves forward, and the elastic in the underwear pulls on the elastic on the resting leg. The non-moving leg is in the stance stage, and here the underwear is pulling on already compressed tissues in the buttocks—causing further compression and damage. So, with every step, you alternatively increase the compression on each buttock. Panty lines should be considered a dangerous weapon in the genesis of dimples on the buttocks. What's worse: the damage is always self-inflicted.

Sleep Naked

In addition to changing underwear style, I recommend that women either sleep naked or wear loose undergarments, because the majority of the lymphatic drainage occurs at night. If you

Tight undergarments are the friends of cellulite. Choose your friends carefully: do not wear this kind of underwear.

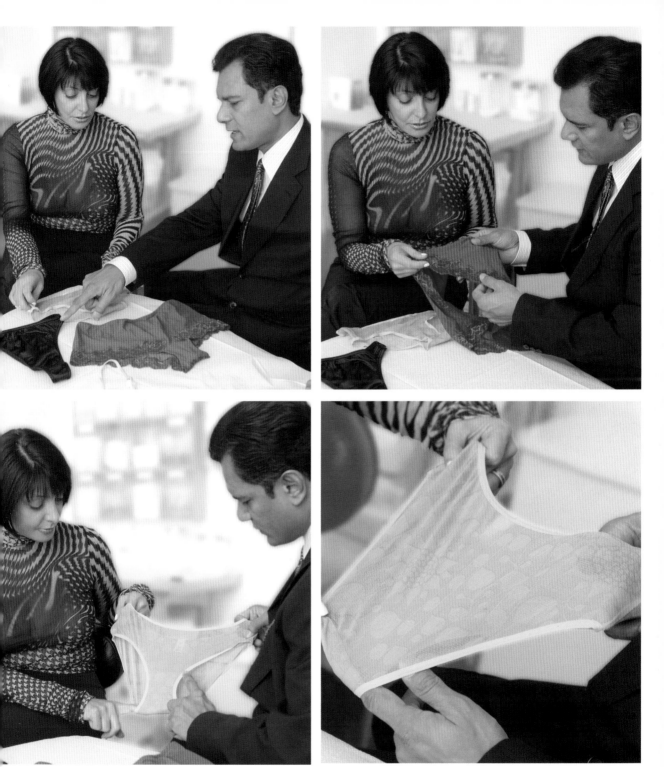

4A–4D: Dr. Bissoon explains the advantages and disadvantages of different underwear. **4A:** Illustrating several underwear styles. **4B:** Lace is better than elastic. **4C & 4D:** Demonstrating the tourniquet-like effect of elastic in underwear across the buttocks.

sleep with underwear that restricts night drainage, you are giving cellulite another helping hand. It's important to wear underwear that doesn't produce panty lines, and it's important to sleep without underwear. If you must sleep with underwear—I know that it gets very cold in some regions—please wear something less constricting.

In my office, I showcase a selection of underwear that is not cellulite friendly. If a woman chooses to continue wearing her usual type of underwear, I recommend that she use such underwear only if it's made from lace instead of elastic. And various styles of underwear made from lace are not difficult to find. The reason I ask for lace is because it doesn't cause panty lines or compress the lymphatic tissues. Making the transition to a G-string or thong is even better, but some women are uncomfortable with this. I never force anyone to adopt a particular style that makes her uncomfortable, so long as the underwear is an enemy of cellulite.

There is only one respect in which underwear that's "tight is all right." That tightness takes the form of compressive stockings. These stockings help prevent and/or retard cellulite formation because they force the lymphatic fluids back from the toes into pelvic circulation. So, I do recommend these stockings. Occasionally, I have seen women wear regular underwear with stockings over them. This is self-defeating, and may produce more harm. Just think: you are applying compression from the legs up when—suddenly—there is a blockage. The cascade is worsened. However, in the summer it can sometimes be too hot to wear such stockings, so don't sweat it—literally.

General Rules for Underwear

1. **_No_** elastic over the buttocks.

2. **_No_** elastic over the inguinal (groin) area.

3. Elastic is okay at the waist.

4. Use underwear with lace instead of elastic.

5. Preferable to wear thongs/G-strings.

6. Not wearing underwear is an option.

7. Stockings/pantyhose is beneficial.

8. Sleep in the nude or a pull-over nighty.

9. Don't wear underwear and pantyhose together.

Puzzled looks appear on the faces of many patients when I explain how panty lines contribute to their dimples. Some appear to be shocked. Others are mildly surprised. Some probably think I've lost my mind. All of them respond by saying, "Nobody ever told me that." That's true. Nobody ever told you that because (until recently) nobody ever studied the phenomenon. I only made the discovery after five years of careful observation. But my conclusions aren't based solely on my own work. There are other scientific findings that lend support to the theory.

In February 1965, Charles Ribaudo, M.D., published an article entitled "Panty Girdle Syndrome" in which he discussed two women he'd evaluated for leg edema. During their evaluations, he observed something curious: both women had a circular skin indentation in the upper thigh. He surmised that the indentations were caused by panty type girdles. Upon his request, the women stopped wearing the garment, and their edema resolved. What Dr. Ribaudo reported was the acute effect of elastic compression on edema formation, which is a step in cellulite formation.

Unfortunately, his work was ignored by underwear manufacturers and scientists alike.

Panty Girdle Syndrome also received attention from Albert Craig, M.D., who published an article, "Constrictive Forces of the Panty Girdle on Thighs," in June 1965. Dr. Craig demonstrated that pressure under the panty girdle increased with sitting, and decreased with standing and walking. He concluded that the force wasn't sufficient to produce edema unless there was damage to the valves in the veins. Craig's observations lend credence to my theory when considered in terms of long-term compression. Elevated, *long-term* compression will result in tissue damage— in the same way that slowly rubbing two sticks together eventually produces fire.

Given all this attention to panty girdles in 1965, you might have expected a flurry of research articles that prompted redesigns of women's underwear. Sadly, this was not the case. More than 30 years passed before another article pointed out the negative effects of tight underwear. Alan Matarasso, M.D. reported on three patients who developed medical complications caused by tight elastic compression over the groin/inguinal area. Two patients developed blood clots beneath the compression sites, and one developed a skin irritation. Although the patients were already at risk, the tight underwear precipitated the complications. Interestingly, Dr. Matarasso called his discovery "Tight Underwear Syndrome" (TUS). TUS can affect both men and women. Men may experience a decrease in sperm count, while women may develop leg edema and (over the long term) dimples across the buttocks.

Tight clothing has many other effects on the body. A study by Yuki Mori and his colleagues demonstrated that tight clothing produces multiple physiological changes. They documented an increase in heart rate, adrenaline, noradrenalin and a significant

increase in nocturnal melatonin.
Subjects who wore tight clothing
tired easily, and movement of their
extremities increased skin compression. The subjects in the tight
clothing group responded as if
they were under stress.

High melatonin levels facilitate
sleep and boost the immune
system. But a 2000 study by
Lee Ya showed that wearing
tight garments at night suppresses
melatonin production—another
reason to sleep naked or in
loose undergarments!

Many scientific papers have
demonstrated the relationship
between acute compression and
physiological changes, some of
which are very subtle. Although

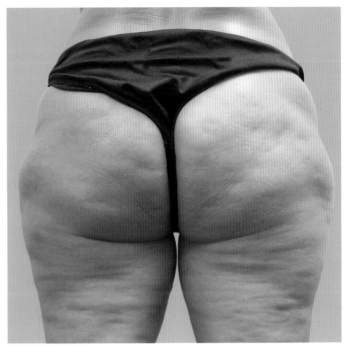

Fig. 5a-5b: This photo illustrates the formation of dimples under the panty lines in this 38 year old woman.
Lionel Bissoon

they may be difficult to perceive, these effects have a cumulative
impact on the body. As the first to observe and report on the
effects of long-term elastic compression over the buttocks,
I advise women concerned about dimples and cellulite to stop
wearing tight undergarments. In my opinion, this is a common
sense measure for preventing the physical, physiological and
cosmetic impact of Panty Line Syndrome on women. ◊

A Letter from "Nicole"

"When I turned 40, I noticed cellulite whenever I would squeeze the skin on my thighs, and I also noticed dimpling on my butt. No matter how much I worked out, the dimples multiplied. The result was that my butt began resembling a mattress. Also, the backs and sides of my upper thighs had deep dimpling, which was noticeable even without 'pinching' the skin.

I dressed to cover my cellulite. By the time I found Dr. Bissoon in September 2003, I hadn't worn a bathing suit in six years. I was mortified at the thought of being seen naked with my cellulite, so I would position myself in such a way that you could not see it. Or I would turn out the lights when making love, even though I prefer soft, romantic lighting. I was obsessed with the way my body looked. I always thought about my cellulite, even when fully dressed. I knew it was there, I was covering it up, and I felt awful about it. When anyone complimented me on how slim I was, I always disputed it, thinking to myself, 'How good could I look? I have this ugly cellulite.'

Every once in a while, I would look at myself in my underwear in front of a mirror, grabbing a handful of butt cheek and say to my mother, 'I need to get rid of this,' but I never said the word 'cellulite.' I could easily discuss my fat: that seemed curable, but the cellulite was an incurable disease that I didn't discuss with anyone.

A Letter from "Nicole" (Continued)

Dr. Bissoon performed Mesotherapy, along with a procedure called Subcision™ on my cellulite.

This treatment was a miracle cure!

I have no cellulite.

I still have to work on 'firming up' and building muscle, but I can actually picture myself wearing a bathing suit again. I know it's a reality, and not a fantasy."

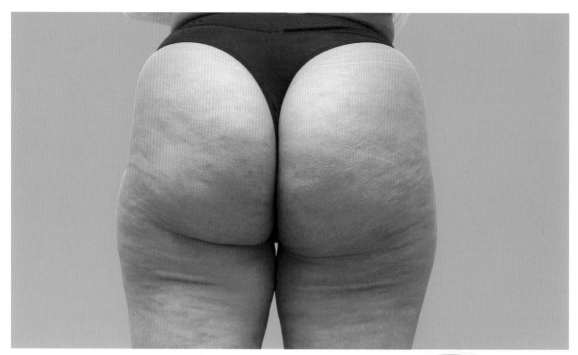

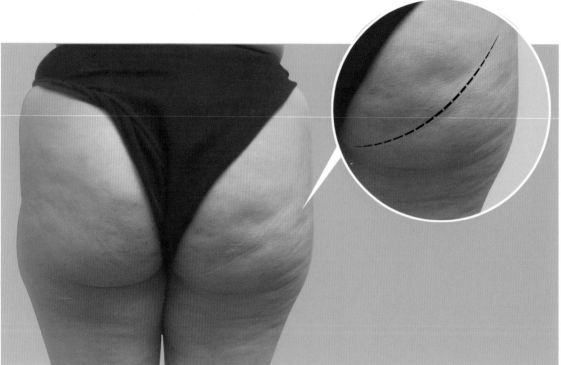

Fig. 6A-6B: A woman with multiple dimples; in the *right* buttock (*bottom*), you can notice the dimple is located under the panty line. She was treated with Subcision™. The photo on the *top* shows the *after* results.

Lionel Bissoon

173 • The Problem with Panties

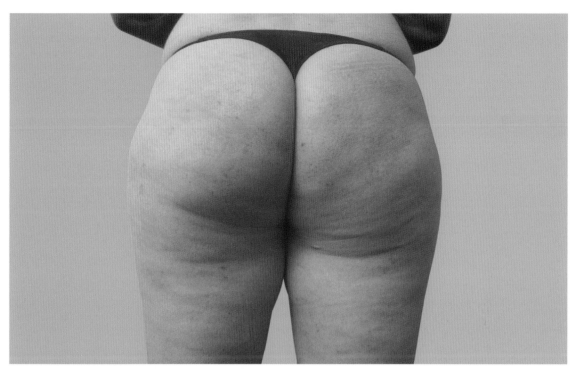
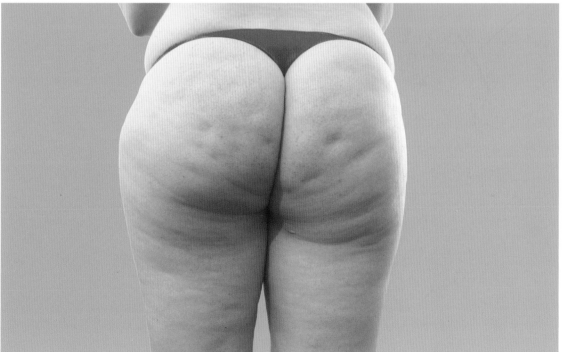

Fig. 7a-7b: This woman was seen for Mesotherapy for her cellulite. Notice the dimples in the buttocks are oriented in the direction of the panty lines. The buttocks were treated with Subcision™, the legs were treated with Mesotherapy *(top)*.

Lionel Bissoon

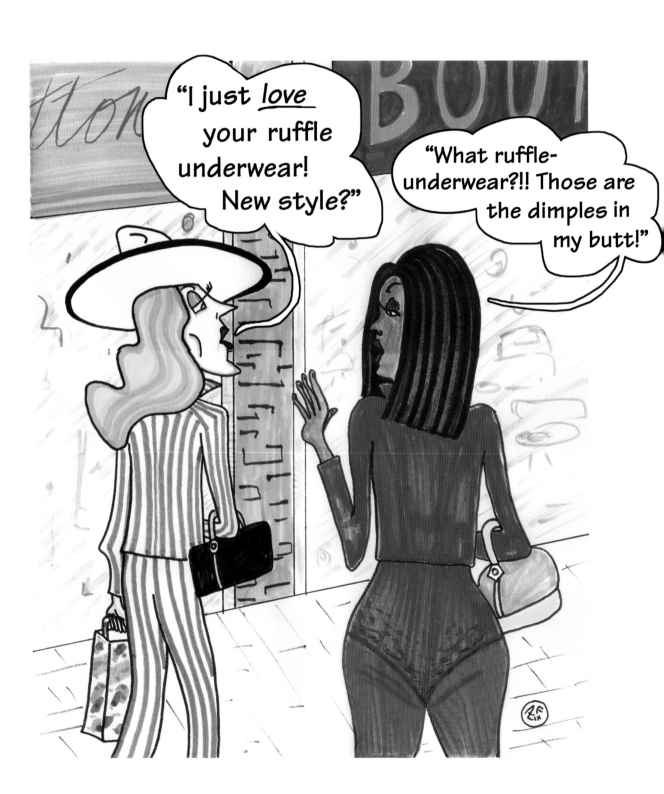

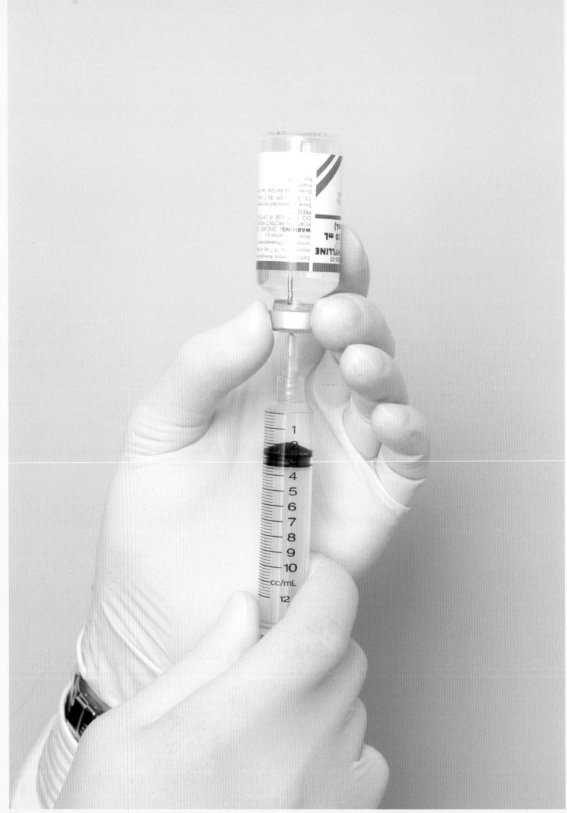

9. *Science and*

Cellulite

Although 90% of women have, or will develop, cellulite

in their lifetimes, many skincare "gurus" such as plastic

surgeons and dermatologists are stumped when asked

about treatments for the disorder. Common responses

include: "liposuction can help," "nobody will notice,"

or most frustrating of all, "you just have to live with it."

The good news is that you don't have to accept these

answers anymore!

Many women believe that cellulite is an untreatable curse. Well, if it's really a curse, then find someone to lift it. One reason so few doctors have aggressively pursued cellulite cures is because no working theory exists about the cause. But knowing the cause doesn't always produce a treatment, and physicians routinely treat conditions without knowing their underlying causes. In these cases, physicians treat the symptoms associated with the disorder. Today's Mesotherapists take this approach by treating the orange peel skin and dimpling associated with cellulite, while simultaneously trying to learn the causes.

Assembling a theory of the origin of cellulite requires information from many disciplines, since there are few published medical treatises on the subject. A recent Medline search turned up approximately 50 articles on cellulite. Of these, roughly 10 had any substance. In this chapter, I'll review these articles, and demonstrate the validity of my theory regarding cellulite formation.

To date, only one article—written by Ana Beatris, R. Rossi and Andre Luiz Vergananini—provides a comprehensive analysis of all the factors involved in the genesis of cellulite. The article quotes works by Alquier and Paviot (published in the 1920s), which describe cellulite as a noninflammatory cellular disorder of mesodermal origin—the result of poor circulation and water metabolism—which extends to the adjacent tissues between cells. The condition was thought to be caused by trauma, infection or a glandular problem. The Vergananini article lists numerous other factors described by various authors. I don't intend to reproduce Vergananini's review of the literature here. I merely want to show how different researchers have contributed to a comprehensive theory of cellulite.

F. Nurnberger, M.D. and G. Muller, M.D. published their landmark article, "So-Called Cellulite: An Invented Disease" in 1978.

Invented? How could a condition experienced by 90% of women be "invented?" Since 1978, too many women have suffered with cellulite because physicians, researchers, husbands, boyfriends and the lay press subscribed to this theory of "invented" cellulite. Nurnberger and Muller's article featured pictures of tissue samples with normal estrogen, lower-than-normal estrogen and an estrogen deficiency. The photos depicting estrogen-deficient tissue show clear evidence of cellulite. Despite this, the authors claimed cellulite was an invented disease. Fortunately, some good came of this report: Mesotherapists use Nurnberger and Muller's grading system to evaluate cellulite.

Too Much Estrogen

One theory of cellulite formation blames excess estrogen. But this theory doesn't explain why women suddenly develop cellulite when entering menopause. Yes, there is a hormonal imbalance, but not of excess estrogen. If excess estrogen were the true culprit, women entering menopause would never develop cellulite. More importantly, if women entering menopause had excess estrogen, there would be no menopause! Estrogen is known to increase collagen synthesis and microcirculation within the skin. This dual action of estrogen may account for the observation that overweight women have excess estrogen, and display little cellulite. So, there's at least one benefit to being overweight!

One can logically conclude that the cellulite formation cascade is initiated with the decrease in estrogen. Once the cascade has started, estrogen replacement will not stop the process, but it will slow the process. Currently, estrogen replacement is controversial, and I don't recommend it for treating cellulite. If you decide to undergo hormone replacement, find a competent physician who is knowledgeable in this area of endocrinology.

Dwindling estrogen triggers a cellulite formation cascade: First, there is a decrease in microcirculation—that is, less blood flows through the small capillaries or vessels to feed the surrounding tissues. Agneta Bergqvist and his colleagues demonstrated that estrogen receptors are present on cells within the peripheral blood vessels (vessels in the arms and legs). These authors also demonstrated the presence of estrogen receptors in the leg veins of fertile women, and that this receptor is absent in some of the leg veins of postmenopausal women. Thus, we can conclude that when estrogen decreases, receptor production also decreases. Once an estrogen decrease is sensed by these cells, they lose their viability, and the capillaries narrow in diameter. In addition, these lifelines for the tissues become fibrotic (inflexible and hard).

Second, the subcutaneous tissues (those lying just under the skin) experience decreased oxygen and nutrition (asphyxia). When this occurs, the fibroblast cells that repair the fibrous connective tissue cannot function effectively. Fibroblasts are important cells involved in both wound healing and tissue repair. They are essential for the continued remodeling of healthy skin. The malfunctioning of fibroblast cells results in weakened and damaged septae. Septae are like the scaffolding supporting a building: they surround and support the lobes of fat cells under the skin.

Third, because of the adverse changes in the maintenance of healthy blood vessels, fluids accumulate within the tissues, and the fat cells become abnormal. The cells become enlarged or hypertrophied, and they protrude by herniating though holes in the septae. The process whereby the fat cells push through the septae is called *herniation*. (See Figures 1 and 2 for examples of herniation and healthy skin.) The fluid accumulation within the tissues causes increased pressure from fluid accumulation, allowing larger fat cells to produce further damage to the already weakened structural support or septae.

We can now summarize the events that occur as a woman approaches menopause and the subsequent formation of cellulite according to the decreased estrogen theory. The first step is a decrease in circulating estrogens. You can logically assume that as estrogens decrease, this leads to adverse changes in the micro-vasculature feeding of the underlying tissues, and causes fibroblasts to malfunction. Fibroblasts do not maintain the septae supporting the fat tissues, and the normal organized morphology (shape of the fat tissues) becomes disorganized due to the movement of fat cells from the lobes of fat.

Indirect support of the low estrogen theory is the observation that estrogen starts to slowly decrease around the ages of 25-35. This age bracket is the same at which many women notice the onset of cellulite, and the process only worsens as they approach menopause. Additionally, there are many studies that have documented increased circulation and increased collagen production in postmenopausal women. When those women were given supplemental estrogen replacements, results indicated an increase in collagen production, fibroblast cell activity, and circulation—and thus decreased the signs of aging in women.

Fluid Retention

Another theory points to increased fluid retention that is secondary to lymphatic and venous insufficiency. This theory is supported by observations of women during pregnancy, as evidenced by the number of women who claim their cellulite developed during pregnancy and continued even after subsequent weight loss. If this theory holds true, every woman with cellulite should eventually develop some degree of lymphaedema and/or peripheral vasculature disease.

Lymphaedema is a scientific term that describes an abnormal accumulation of the nutrient- and oxygen-depleted fluid that

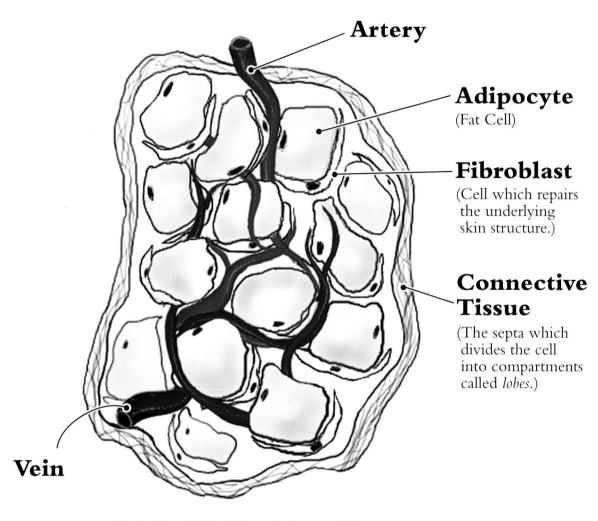

Artery

Adipocyte
(Fat Cell)

Fibroblast
(Cell which repairs
the underlying
skin structure.)

**Connective
Tissue**
(The septa which
divides the cell
into compartments
called *lobes*.)

Vein

*Lobule of Healthy Adipose Tissue
Showing Maintenance of Tissue Integrity*

Fig. 1: Healthy Adipose Tissue

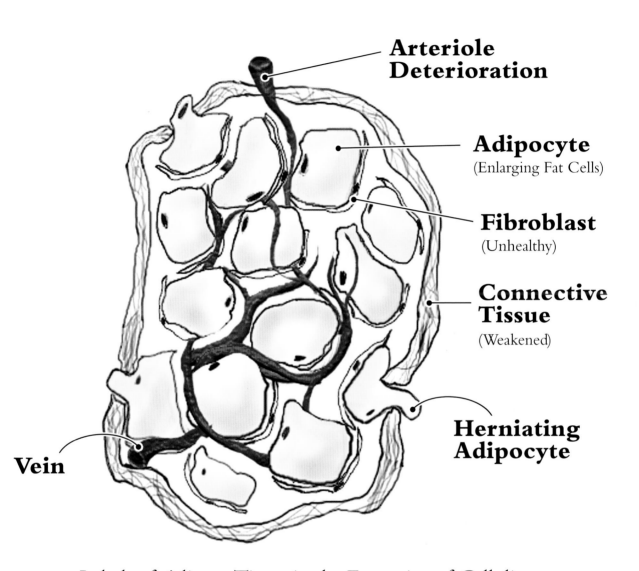

Arteriole Deterioration

Adipocyte
(Enlarging Fat Cells)

Fibroblast
(Unhealthy)

Connective Tissue
(Weakened)

Herniating Adipocyte

Vein

Lobule of Adipose Tissue in the Formation of Cellulite

Fig. 2: Tissue Showing Cellulite Formation

drains from tissues. While this theory may hold true for some women, I don't believe it's the primary cause of cellulite.

A study performed using Magnetic Resonance Imaging (MRI) to evaluate the water content in women with cellulite revealed no evidence of abnormal fluid retention within the cellulite. It's my belief, however, that some form of lymphatic stasis contributes to cellulite. By lymphatic stasis, I'm referring to a lack of fluid movement or drainage from tissues due to chronic compression across the buttocks and inguinal (inner thigh) areas. The compression is caused by:

A. Elastic underwear

B. Prolonged sitting

C. Sitting with legs crossed

Deposition of Amino-Sugar Complexes

In another article, T. Lotti, M.D. and colleagues evaluated tissue samples or biopsies from cadavers with cellulite. The study revealed increased concentrations of glycosaminoglycans, which are half-sugar, half-amino-acid that behave like sticky glue. Three flavors of glycosaminoglycans—dermatan dextran sulfate, chondroitin sulfate and hyaluronic acid—were found. These molecules are responsible for the water retained in cellulite.

Other studies have revealed deposits of glycosaminoglycans in aging skin, but there seem to be larger concentrations in cellulitic tissues. The only possible mechanism by which I can explain this phenomenon is that the formation of glycosaminoglycans is secondary to lymphatic damage, and that the precipitation and concentration of these molecules occurs within already-damaged tissues. Hence, if one could break up and remove these complex molecules from the local tissue, this could facilitate tissue repair. Lotti and his colleagues exposed cellulite tissues to three different enzymes that break up glycosaminoglycans, and examined the tissues under a microscope. The cellulite tissue appeared normal after the enzymatic treatment. One of the enzymes employed was hyaluronidase, which is used in Mesotherapy to treat cellulite.

An article by B. Querleux, which evaluated cellulite using MRI, showed no increase of water in the interstitial spaces (between cells). Although I place credence in these findings, the report doesn't explain the increased amounts of hyaluronate, dextran sulfate and chondroitin sulfate found in cellulite. The only explanation is that microscopic amounts of fluid and glycosaminoglycans are leaking across the vascular cell membranes from the capillary side. We know that there are fenestrations (microscopic pores or holes) in the dermal capillaries, and that these pores allow some fluid molecules to freely diffuse across the vascular membranes. The large molecules that diffuse across these membranes do not enter the lymphatic and venous capillaries, but they do precipitate in the skin because of the poorly functioning fibroblast cells. The water or edema is trapped in the glycoproteins, and thus cannot be seen by MRI.

All of this prompts a major question on cellulite formation: Why does cellulite seem to first occur in the buttocks, lateral thighs and around the knees? Remember, anatomists know there are three layers of fat in these areas of a woman's body: the subcutaneous fat, steatometry (or middle fat layer) and the deep fat reserve. These layers are more responsive to hormones when storing fat during pregnancy and starvation. But today, a woman with cellulite isn't necessarily starving or pregnant.

My Conclusions

I can only conclude that the initial causative factor in cellulite genesis is the decrease in circulating estrogen. A major contributing environmental factor to cellulite formation and dimpling is static fluid accumulation within cellulitic tissues, due to environmental factors such as constrictive undergarments. I have proposed this theory in the hopes that it will be tested and evaluated through research. The goal of the research is the long-term maintenance of healthy, smooth and attractive skin, as well as body sculpting. This is my theory. Whether it will be supported through continued research remains to be determined.

What's important is that Mesotherapists continue to effectively treat the symptoms of cellulite, regardless of the theory's validity. Right or wrong, the treatable factors remain constant. Hence, the real focus of this book is the proper treatment of cellulite. Although it's great to have a better understanding of the underlying causes, the ultimate goal of medicine is to improve the patient's physical and psychological condition.

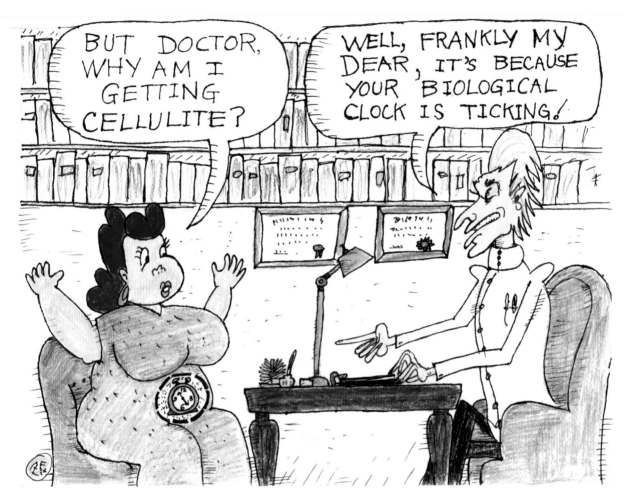

Fig. 3: Dr. Dred explains the cause of cellulite to Cellulina.

A Letter from "Nancy" • February 22, 2003

"Two years ago I went for a consultation regarding Liposuction. I was determined to get rid of my fat thighs and lose the ripples from my butt. The doctor told me she could reduce the inside of my thighs…but the appearance of the skin would be the same. I told her I had to think about it, and left feeling very depressed.

I'm only five-feet tall, so my legs and butt have always been the biggest part of me. I have always had to exercise, diet and watch what I eat to maintain a decent shape. When I was in my late 30s, I noticed the texture of my thighs and butt changing—to the point where I couldn't stand to look at myself in the mirror.

Six months later, I saw a news segment showing Dr. Bissoon treating a patient with injections for **cellulite**. I went online, performed a Google search, and immediately called Dr. Bissoon.

On my first visit, Dr. Bissoon explained what his therapy involved, and what I could expect my legs to look like after 8–10 sessions. He took pictures and did a patch test to make sure I wouldn't have an allergic reaction. Then he told me **to never again wear the type of underwear I'd been wearing**. He told me that it cuts off the circulation, and (as it turned out) the area he talked about is exactly where I had the largest dimples.

A Letter from "Nancy" • February 22, 2003 (Continued)

After three Mesotherapy sessions, there was a noticeable difference. You couldn't see ripples through my pants anymore, and I could wear tighter pants again.

I've had about 10 treatments, including a Subcision™ treatment for the deep pockets on the backs of my thighs. I haven't missed any time from work, which was another factor that made this so easy. Although I'm still healing from the Subcision™ treatment, the deep pockets are gone: very hard to believe! When Dr. Bissoon shows me my "before" pictures, I can't believe I used to look like that. I still have trouble looking at them. They're horrifying.

I can't say much more, except that I love Dr. Bissoon and what he's done for me. When there are patients in the clinic that are 'iffy' about having the procedure done, I have not only asked if they wanted to see my 'before' pictures, I've actually pulled down my pants to show them what I look like now!"

Sincerely,

Nancy
Cooper City, Florida

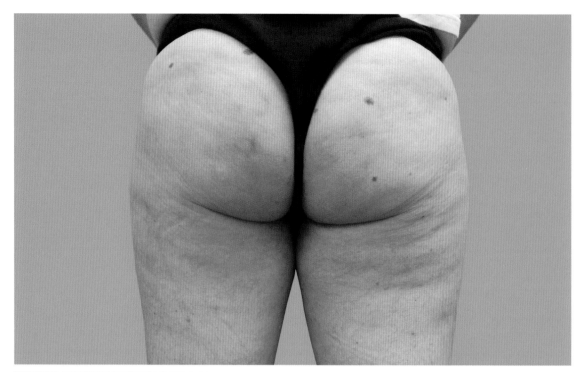

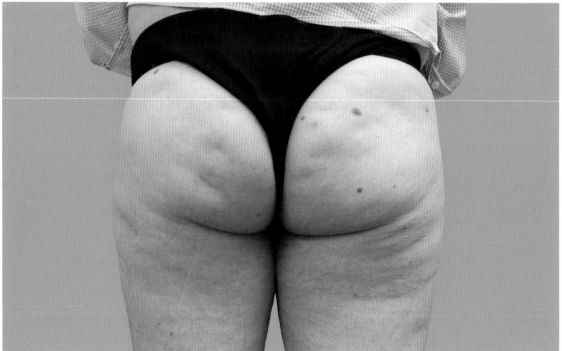

Fig. 4A-4B: It is commonly thought that men do not have cellulite. This series of photographs show a male patient who was treated with Subcision™/Stringcision™ and Mesotherapy.

Lionel Bissoon

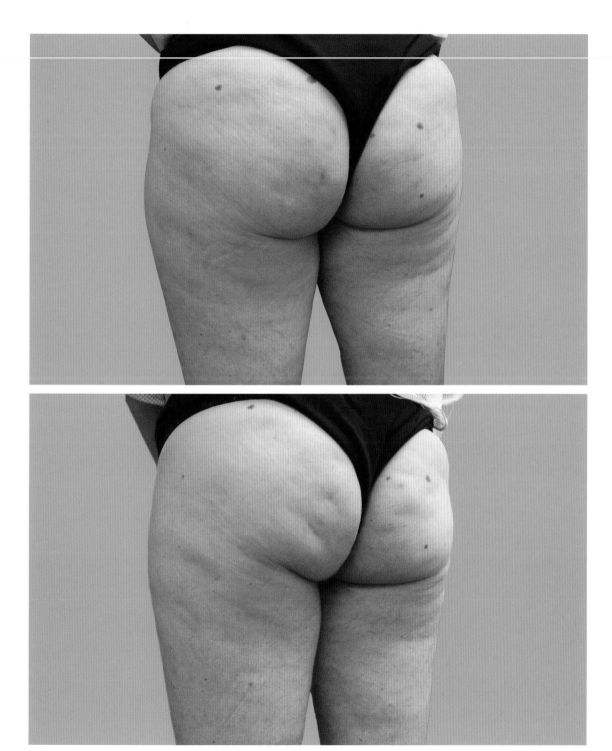

Fig. 5a-5b: This is a three-quarters view of the buttock of the man *before (bottom)* and *after (top)*.
Lionel Bissoon

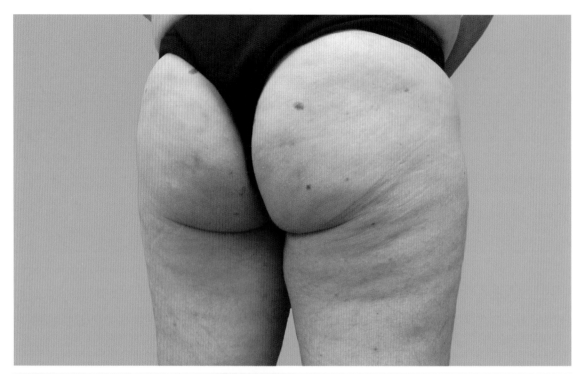

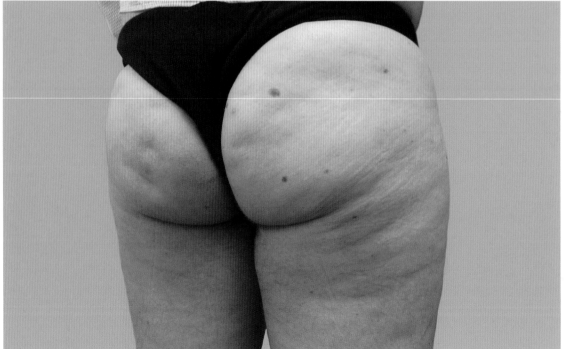

FIG. 6A-6B: This is another three-quarters view of the man.

Lionel Bissoon

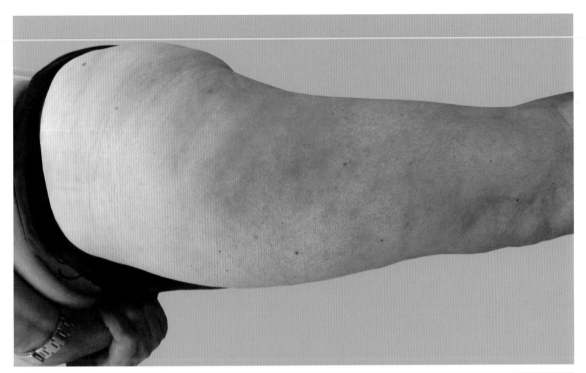

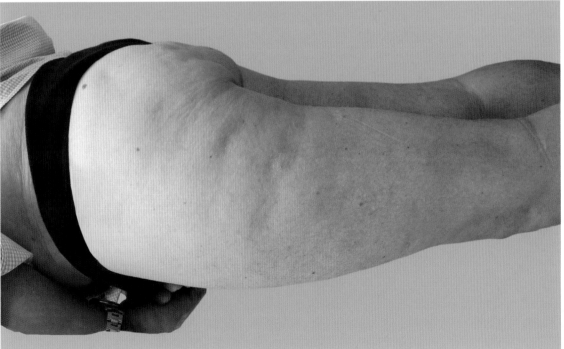

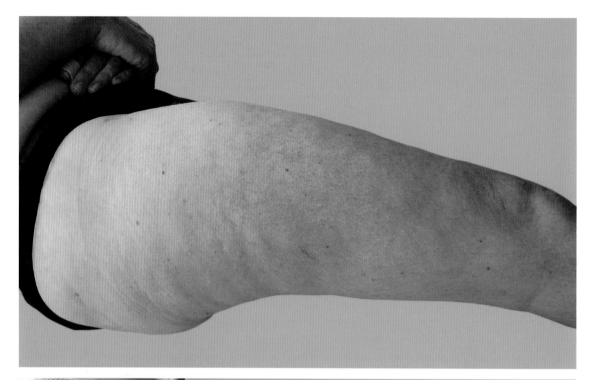

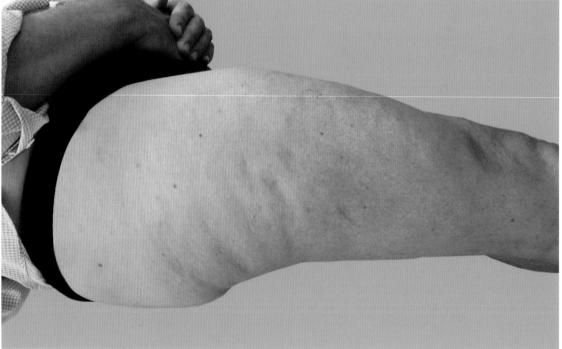

Fig. 8A-8B Same Patient.

Lionel Bissoon

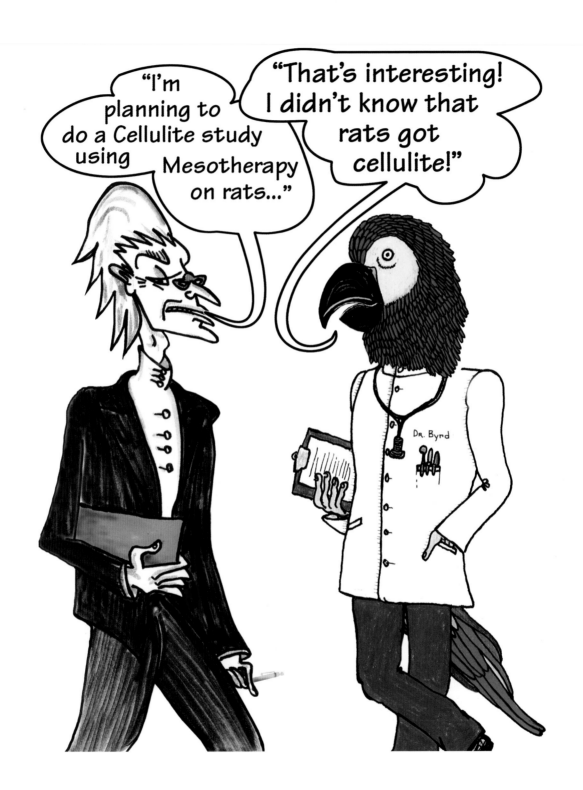

75¢

New York Herald

Crown Newspapers

Local Forecast: Blustery, clouds, highs in the 40s, winds out of the north, 50% chance of precipitation

VOLUME 163   NEW YORK, TUESDAY, FEBRUARY 12, 2006   SEVENTY FIVE CENTS

Your Weather Forecast
Page 27

MESOTHERAPY OK'D

Residents of NY Get Flu Vaccine

City adds elderly to flu program

In the state of New York, many elderly, children and people with compromised immune systems get the flu each winter season. Estimates conclude that as many as 2,000 die from flu outbreaks. Sadly, most of these deaths should be preventable—especially if the vaccine is available and public education and programs are functioning.

For those of highest risk and age 65 and over, that annual flu shot is *the* best way to prevent the most severe complications of the flu. The flu shot is safe and will

Sports News
New York Pumas Stats

TEAM STATISTICS				
	PTS	YDS	RUSH	PASS
OFFENSE	20.3	340.9	147.2	193.7
DEFENSE	15.3	293.3	101.3	192.0

INDIVIDUAL LEADERS				
PASSING	ATT	COMP	YDS	TD
DiAngelo	334	221	2492	15
DiAngelo	CAR	YDS	AVG	TD
Smythe	343	1544	5	12.0
Bernis	86	456	5	2.0
RECEIVING	REC	YDS	AVG	TD
Mcavoy	41	810	20	5.0
Quartovento	50	708	14	4.0

Complete Team statistics | Roster

2006 AFC EAST STANDINGS

TEAM	W	L	T	HM	RD	PF	PA
New England	13	2	0	7-0	6-2	416	253
New York	10	5	0	6-2	4-3	304	229
Buffalo	9	6	0	5-2	4-4	371	255
Miami	4	11	0	3-5	1-6	252	324

Complete Standings

Coalition Forces in Iraq Increase

Insurgents Open Fire

By Gene Feinmann

Coalition forces have increased on the ground in both Baghdad and other parts of the country as pressure has mounted from insurgents. Coalition troops will have an increasingly difficult and dangerous drives from any two points in the country and especially as they go through Iraq's capital city, Baghdad.

Military analysts weighed in this week on the future of an increasingly dangerous ground war. Retired U.S. Army Brig. Gen. David Grainis and retired U.S. Air Force Maj. Gen. Lon Shepperd have said that complications of

Surgeon General: "Mesotherapy does not need FDA approval..."

By Sara Bellum
Staff Writer

In a startling statement today both in the ABC affiliates and as reported earlier in discussions spun off from the *New England Journal of Medicine*, the United States Surgeon General acknowledged that Mesotherapy "does not need, nor did it ever need FDA approval." The news is bounding both in the popular press and in medical journals, due in part to increased awareness and popularity of this technique spawned by the national best-seller *The Cellulite Cure*, by Dr. Lionel Bissoon.

Mr. Hutt, the former FDA Chief Counsel and noted legal authority, was quoted as saying "FDA has no statutory authority whatever to ap

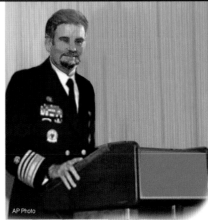

AP Photo

The Surgeon General today at a press conference on Mesotherapy

10. *Mesotherapy and the*
FDA

When discussing Mesotherapy, the issue of FDA

approval is usually raised. I have had to explain the role

of the FDA regarding Mesotherapy to a number of

journalists. Invariably, the writer or broadcaster simply

announces that Mesotherapy "does not have FDA

approval." That is true, but it fails to reflect the fact

that FDA is not responsible for approving medical

and surgical procedures.

Since so many people have a negative reaction to the phrase "does not have FDA approval," I have included this chapter on the FDA's history and responsibilities, as well as its relationship specifically with Mesotherapy and its practitioners.

In May 2004, former FDA Chief Counsel Peter Barton Hutt spoke at a seminar sponsored by The Bissoon Institute of Mesotherapy. Mr. Hutt is a partner in the Washington, D.C. law firm of Covington and Burling specializing in food and drug law. He graduated from Yale College and Harvard Law School and obtained a Master of Laws degree from NYU Law School. Mr. Hutt served as Chief Counsel for the Food and Drug Administration during 1971–1975. He is the co-author of the casebook used to teach food and drug law throughout the country. Since 1994 he has taught a full course on this subject during the Winter Term at Harvard Law School, and he taught the same course during the Spring Term at Stanford Law School in 1998. Mr. Hutt has been a member of the Institute of Medicine since it was founded in 1971. He serves on academic and venture capital advisory boards, and the boards of startup biotechnology companies. He currently serves on the Panel on the Administrative Restructuring of the National Institutes of Health. He was named by the *Washingtonian* magazine as one of Washington's 50 best lawyers (out of 40,000) and as one of Washington's 100 most influential people; by the National Law Journal as one of the 40 best health care lawyers in the United States; and by the European Counsel as the best FDA regulatory specialist in Washington, D.C. Business Week referred to Mr. Hutt in June 2003 as the "unofficial dean of Washington food and drug lawyers."

After the meeting, I asked Mr. Hutt if he would consent to an interview on FDA issues, so that patients and physicians can understand the authority of FDA to regulate drugs and medical devices and the relationship of this authority to the practice of Mesotherapy. The following is the interview with Mr. Hutt. See Figure 2.

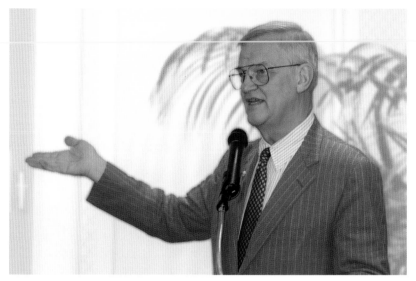

Dr. Bissoon: What was the origin of the Food and Drug Administration?

Mr. Hutt: Every recorded civilization has enacted some form of controls over the food and drug supply. These types of laws were brought to our country by our earliest settlers. Thus, the origin of food and drug law in the United States is as old as the country itself.

In our early days, food and drug laws were enacted by cities, counties, and states. There was no federal control, because the regulation of the manufacture and sale of products was thought to be a matter for local, not national, jurisdiction. Indeed, until 1900—when the United States Supreme Court began to recognize that our rapidly-developing commerce required federal as well as state controls—all regulation of food and drugs remained at the local level. In the mid–1800s, the United States Patent Office

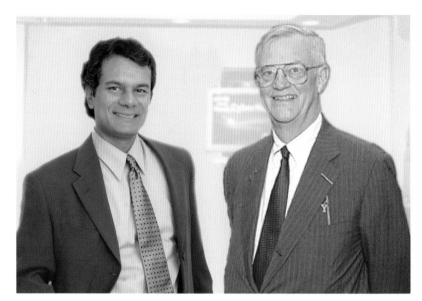

Fig. 2: Dr. Bissoon meets with Mr. Hutt.
© Steven Ladner

Mr. Hutt
(Continued)

established an Agricultural Division and, within it, a chemical laboratory, in order to evaluate claims made in agricultural patents. When Congress established the United States Department of Agriculture in 1862, the Agricultural Division and its chemical laboratory became the nucleus of the new department. The laboratory was renamed the Chemical Division and later, in 1902, the Bureau of Chemistry. It became the Food, Drug, and Insecticide Administration in 1927 and assumed its current name, the Food and Drug Administration, in 1930. FDA remained a part of USDA until 1939, when it was transferred to the Federal Security Agency. In 1953 the Federal Security Agency was incorporated into the Department of Health, Education, and Welfare, and in 1979 that Department was reorganized as the Department of Health and Human Services. Thus, FDA today is part of the Department of Health and Human

Services, along with such other health agencies as the National Institutes of Health, the Centers for Disease Control and Prevention, the Centers for Medicare and Medicaid Services, and the Public Health Service.

Dr. Bissoon: When did federal regulation of pharmaceutical products begin?

Mr. Hutt: The first bill to regulate pharmaceutical products on a national level was introduced in Congress in 1789. It took twenty-seven years of hearings and debate before that bill became law as the Federal Food and Drug Act of 1906. The 1906 Act authorized FDA to regulate food and drugs, but not cosmetics and medical devices. When Franklin Delano Roosevelt became President in 1933, FDA convinced him that the 1906 Act should be modernized. This time it took five years of congressional hearings and debate before Congress enacted the Federal Food, Drug, and Cosmetic Act (FD&C Act) of 1938. Since that law was enacted, it has been amended more than one hundred times. The FD&C Act, as it is amended today, is extremely long, complex, and very difficult to understand.

Dr. Bissoon: What types of products does FDA regulate under the FD&C Act of 1938?

Mr. Hutt: FDA regulates food (including animal feed), human drugs (including non-prescription and prescription products), animal drugs (including non-prescription and prescription products), biological products (such as vaccines and blood), medical devices, and cosmetics. Focusing on drugs, it is important to understand that any product that is represented to prevent or treat disease, or to affect the structure or function of the human body, comes within the statutory definition of a drug. Any similar claims made for any instrument, apparatus, implement, machine, or similar article will result in the product being classified as a medical device. If an article is represented only to promote personal attractiveness or to alter appearance, but not to affect the structure or function of the body, it is classified as a cosmetic. The FDA statutory authority for regulating drugs and devices is very stringent, and requires either pre-market review or pre-market approval. The FDA statutory authority over cosmetics is more limited, but is nonetheless sufficient to assure that cosmetics are safe and properly labeled.

Dr. Bissoon: It is clear that FDA regulates both the drugs and the devices that are used in Mesotherapy. Does FDA have statutory authority to regulate the procedures and techniques used by physicians in the practice of medicine?

Mr. Hutt: No. FDA has no statutory authority whatever to approve or disapprove medical techniques and procedures, such as those used by physicians in the practice of surgery or Mesotherapy, or to regulate these medical specialty areas in any other way. FDA has repeatedly said it has no direct power of any kind over the practice of medicine. Physicians are therefore free to practice

Mesotherapy without any form of FDA approval for any medical technique or practice area—even if asked to do so.

Dr. Bissoon: Does FDA participate in any way in the licensure of physicians?

Mr. Hutt: No. The licensure of physicians is controlled by state law, not by federal law, and FDA therefore has no role in this area.

Dr. Bissoon: Can FDA restrict or prohibit a physician from practicing medicine or surgery?

Dr. Hutt: No. FDA can prohibit the use of a drug or device, but once that drug or device is lawfully marketed in the United States any state-licensed physician is authorized to use it. FDA cannot revoke or limit in any way a state license to practice medicine.

Dr. Bissoon: You have said that FDA can prohibit the use of a drug. Please explain this.

Mr. Hutt: Under the FD&C Act, no drug may lawfully be imported from abroad, or manufactured in the United States (with extremely limited exceptions), without FDA approval. In order to obtain that approval, the sponsor of the new drug must first investigate the drug under an investigational new drug (IND) application and then submit to FDA and obtain approval of a new drug application (NDA). This is an extremely lengthy, complex, and costly procedure. Thus, as a general rule, any drug must have an approved NDA before a physician can use it in the United States.

As I noted, there are a few limited exceptions. A few old drugs for which no NDA was ever obtained prior to 1962 still remain on the market without formal FDA approval, under an FDA Compliance Policy Guide that permits continued marketing. It is also possible, although extremely difficult, to make a drug wholly within a single state, using machinery that comes only from within that state, and to use it only on patients residing in that state—resulting only in intrastate commerce, which is regulated by the state rather than by FDA. These are, however, unusual exceptions.

Dr. Bissoon: Once FDA approves a drug, how does FDA regulate it?

Mr. Hutt: Following approval of an NDA, the drug may be lawfully marketed throughout the United States. FDA retains substantial surveillance over the marketing of the product to make certain that its labeling continues to reflect the most recent information on safety and effectiveness. FDA retains the authority to withdraw approval of the drug if the agency concludes that the drug is no longer shown to be safe or effective or if it is being improperly manufactured.

Dr. Bissoon: What are the limits placed on physicians in using a drug for which FDA has approved an NDA?

Mr. Hutt: **FDA adopted a policy in 1972, and has reiterated it many times since then, that a physician has the lawful right to prescribe any FDA-approved drug for an unapproved use, as part of the**

practice of medicine. Thus, a physician is not bound in any way by the drug package insert approved by the agency as part of the NDA process. FDA explicitly recognizes that a physician may prescribe an approved drug under any condition that falls outside the approved package insert, without violating the FD&C Act. For example, the drug may be prescribed or used by a physician for a completely different indication, or at a different dosage level, or using a different method of administration, or contrary to a warning or contraindication set forth in the labeling, if the physician concludes that this best serves the interest of the individual patient.

There are, of course, other non–FDA societal controls that could apply if a physician prescribed or used an approved drug for an unapproved use that could not possibly be defended as medically reasonable. State licensing authorities have the power to withdraw the physician's license to practice medicine. A medical institution may withdraw permission for the physician to practice medicine in that particular institution. Patients may also bring malpractice suits, claiming damages.

Dr. Bissoon: As I understand it, you have said that a physician does not violate the FD&C Act by prescribing or using an approved drug for an unapproved use, but does violate the FD&C Act by using an unapproved drug for any use. Is that correct?

Mr. Hutt: That is absolutely correct. It is extremely important for physicians to understand these two basic rules.

Dr. Bissoon:	Does it make any difference whether a drug is imported from abroad or is available here in the United States?
Mr. Hutt:	No. Imported and domestic drugs are treated identically under the FD&C Act.
Dr. Bissoon:	For centuries, pharmacists have compounded drugs on the order of a physician for an individual patient. How is this regulated by FDA?
Mr. Hutt:	FDA has established a policy that recognizes the right of a pharmacist to compound a drug, on the order of a physician for an individual patient, using active ingredients that have been approved for use in the United States under an NDA. It is unlawful, however, for a pharmacist to compound a drug using an active ingredient that has not been approved under an NDA for any purpose.

There are limits on compounding pharmacists. FDA has stated that the following factors will be considered in determining when a compounding pharmacist steps over the line and becomes an illegal drug manufacturer:

- Compounding drugs in anticipation of receiving prescriptions.

- Compounding drugs that have been withdrawn or removed from the market for safety reasons.

- Compounding finished drugs using active ingredients that have not been made in an FDA-registered facility.

- Using drug components that do not meet official compendia requirements.

- Using commercial scale manufacturing.

- Compounding drugs for third parties who resell them.

- Compounding drugs that are commercially available in the marketplace.

- Failing to operate in conformance with state pharmacy law.

If a pharmacist only compounds drugs using active ingredients that have been approved by FDA for some purpose in an existing NDA, and in response to a physician's prescription for an individual patient, none of these problems should occur.

Dr. Bissoon: Can physicians compound medications in their own office for use in Mesotherapy?

Mr. Hutt: The same rules apply to physicians as to pharmacists. Physicians can therefore compound drugs, using approved active ingredients, for use by an individual patient.

Dr. Bissoon: Is there any limit on a pharmacist or physician combining more than one active ingredient in a compounded drug?

Mr. Hutt: No. As long as each active ingredient is approved by FDA under an NDA for some use in the United States, it may be included in a compounded combination drug. There is no limit on the number of drugs that can be included in a lawfully compounded product.

Dr. Bissoon:	Can a pharmaceutical company promote unapproved uses of an approved new drug?
Mr. Hutt:	As a general rule, this is prohibited. Pharmaceutical companies can directly promote only the uses of a drug that are explicitly approved by FDA in the package insert for that drug. It is illegal for a pharmaceutical company to promote its approved drugs for any unapproved uses.
	Pharmaceutical companies can, under limited circumstances, educate physicians about unapproved uses of approved new drugs. The company can respond to a physician's questions with accurate and non-misleading information. Reprints of peer-reviewed medical journal articles can, in appropriate circumstances, be provided to physicians. But direct promotion of an approved drug for an unapproved use is unlawful.
Dr. Bissoon:	Let me turn now to medical devices. How are these products regulated by FDA?
Mr. Hutt:	Under the medical device provisions of the FD&C Act, there are two ways for a new medical device to be introduced into the United States market, whether imported or made domestically. First, a manufacturer may submit a pre-market notification for a medical device to FDA under Section 510(k) of the FD&C Act, demonstrating that the device is substantially equivalent to a previously marketed device that was also subject to a pre-market notification. These submissions are usually

referred to as a "510(k)" submission. FDA reviews a 510(k) submission and clears the device for a specific use. More than ninety eight percent of medical devices are cleared for marketing under this procedure.

For a few truly new medical devices, the FD&C Act requires submission and approval of a pre-market approval (PMA) application, which is similar to the NDA procedure used for new drugs. It is a more complex and lengthy procedure than the 510(k) procedure and is therefore used only where significant issues of safety or effectiveness are involved.

Dr. Bissoon: Are there any exceptions to these two types of FDA review and approval of medical devices?

Mr. Hutt: Yes. For the simplest of medical device— e.g., crutches and tongue depressors—the FDA has created an exemption even from 510(k) clearance. More important for physicians, however, is a statutory exemption for what are called "custom" devices. An individual physician may obtain a specially-made custom medical device, that has not gone through any of the FDA clearance processes, if it is intended to meet the special needs of the physician for use in medical practice and is not generally available to or used by other physicians. This is a narrow exception. It does not apply where a device manufacturer makes a medical device and then sells it to a number of physicians. It must be tailored to the individual physician and otherwise not generally available.

Dr. Bissoon:	What if a physician wishes to use an FDA-cleared medical device for a purpose that falls outside the FDA-approved labeling?
Mr. Hutt:	The same FDA policy that applies to unapproved uses of approved new drugs also applies to unapproved uses of approved medical devices. The physician may use any medical device that is lawfully marketed in the United States for an unapproved use, without violating the FD&C Act. If a device is not approved for any medical use in the United States, however, no physician may lawfully use it for such a purpose.
Dr. Bissoon:	What must a physician do in order to use a completely unapproved drug or device?
Mr. Hutt:	The FD&C Act explicitly provides for investigational use of an unapproved drug or device. For a drug, the physician must submit to FDA an IND application. For a device, the physician must submit to FDA an investigational device exemption (IDE) application. In most instances, these applications are submitted by manufacturers rather than by individual physicians, because they are complex and lengthy documents. Individual physicians are, however, fully entitled to make these types of submissions, and in fact individual investigators often do so.
Dr. Bissoon:	To summarize, it would appear that there is substantial flexibility in the legitimate medical practice of Mesotherapy as long as approved drugs and devices are used.

Mr. Hutt: Yes. As long as the physician or compounding pharmacist begins with active ingredients that have been approved by FDA under an NDA for some use in the United States, the physician has the right to use those drugs in a different combination, at different dosage levels, and for different uses than FDA has approved. Lawfully marketed medical devices can similarly be used in whatever way the physician believes is most appropriate for the individual patient. It is only unapproved drugs and devices that cannot be used. ◊

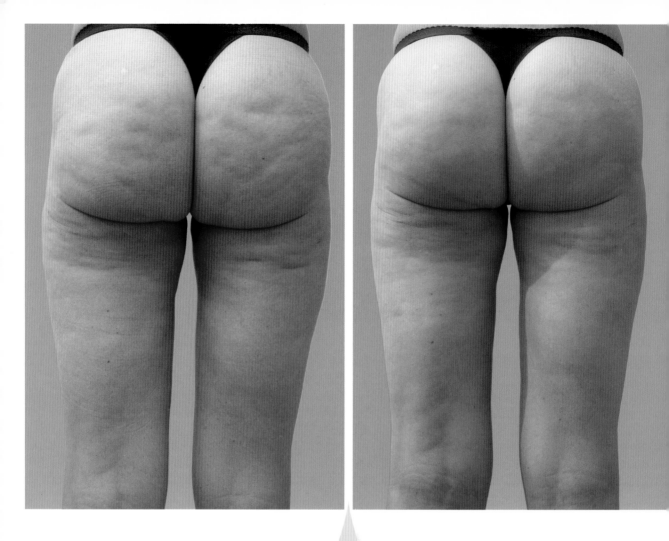

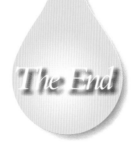

The End

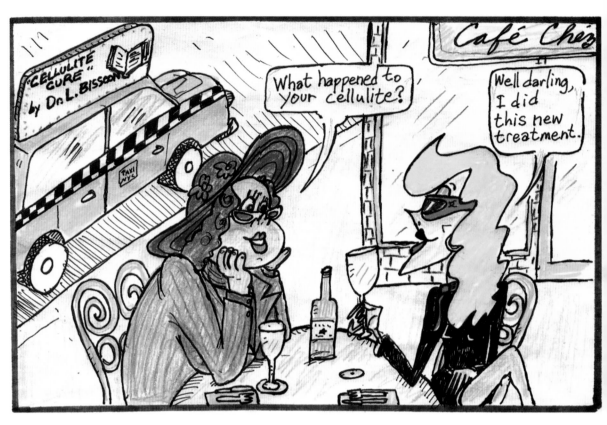

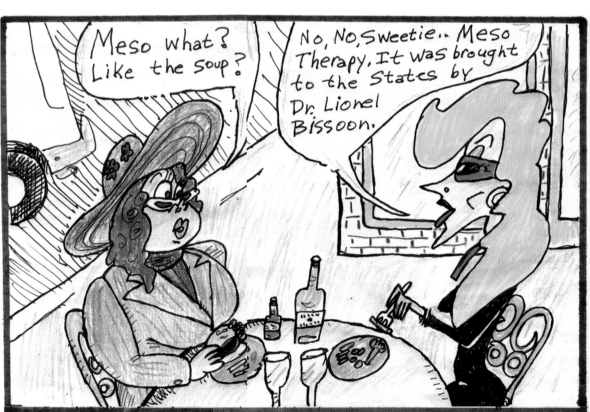

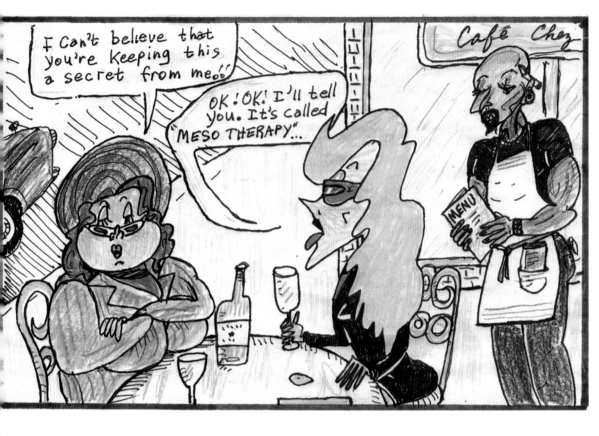

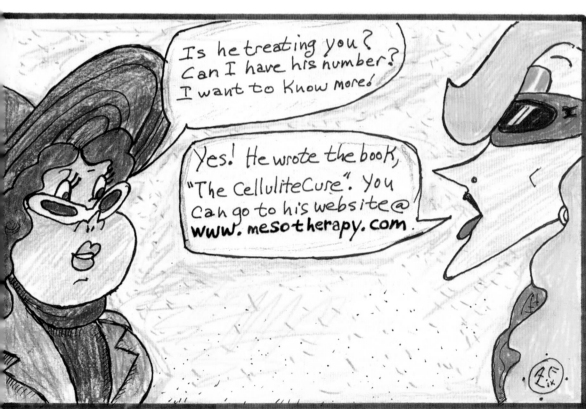

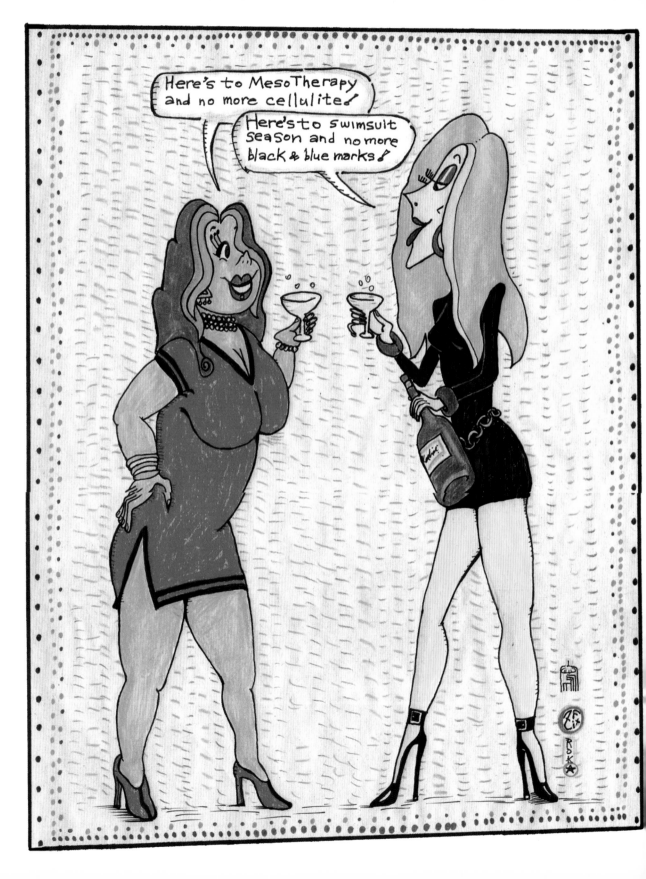

Suggested Reading

Bergqvist A., Bergqvist D., Ferno M. "Estrogen and progesterone receptors in vessel walls. Biochemical and immunochemical assays." *Acta Obstet Gynecol Scand.* January 1993; 72(1): 10-6.

Bertin C., Zunino H., Pittet J.C., Beau P., Pineau P., Massonneau M., Robert C., Hopkins J. "A double-blind evaluation of the activity of an anti-cellulite product containing retinol, caffeine, and ruscogenine by a combination of several non-invasive methods." *J Cosmet Sci.* July-August 2001; 52(4): 199-210.

"Cellulite meltdown?" *Harv. Womens Health Watch.* August 1998; 5 (12): 7.

Cid M.C., Schnaper H.W., Kleinman H.K. "Estrogens and the vascular endothelium." *Ann NY Acad Sci.* June 2002; 966: 143-57.

Collis N., Elliot L.A., Sharpe C., Sharpe D.T. "Cellulite treatment: a myth or reality: a prospective randomized, controlled trial of two therapies, endermologie and aminophylline cream." *Plast Reconstr Surg.* September 1999; 104(4): 1110-4; discussion 1115-7.

Craig Jr., Albert B., M.D. and Dvorak, Maria. "Constrictive Forces of Panty Girdle on Thigh." *New York State Journal of Medicine.* June 1, 1965; 1338.

Critser, Greg. *Fat Land.* Boston: Houghton-Mifflin Co, 2003.

Dancey, Elisabeth, M.D. *The Cellulite Solution.* New York: St. Martin's Press, 1997.

Draelos Z.D., Marenus K.D. "Cellulite. Etiology and purported treatment." *Dermatol Surg.* December 1997; 23(12): 1177-81.

Ersek RA., Mann G.E. 2nd, Salisbury S., Salisbury AV. "Noninvasive mechanical body contouring: a preliminary clinical outcome study." *Aesthetic Plast Surg.* March-April 1997; 21(2): 61-7.

Farhat M.Y., Abi-Younes S., Ramwell P.W. "Non-genomic effects of estrogen and the vessel wall." *Biochem Pharmacol.* March 1996 8; 51(5): 571-6.

Garcia, Oz. *Look and Feel Fabulous Forever.* New York: Harper-Collins Publishers Inc., 2002.

Gharib S. *Harv Health Lett.* August 2003; 28(10): 8.

Grazer, F.M., de Jong, R.H., "Fatal outcomes from liposuction: consensus survey of cosmetic surgeons." *Plast. Reconstr. Surg.* January 2000; 105(1):436-46; discussion 447-8.

Greenwood-Robinson, Maggie, Ph.D. *The Cellulite Breakthrough.* New York: Dell Publishing, 2000.

Greenway, Frank L., Abray, George A., and Heber, David. "Topical Fat Reduction." *Obesity Research.* November 1995: 561S-568S.

Hauser, Ross A., M.D., and Hauser, Marion A., M.S., R.D. *Treating Cancer with Insulin Potentiation Therapy.* Oak Park, Illinois: Beulah Land Press, 2002.

Hexsel, Doris Maria, M.D., and Mazzuco, Rosemari, M.D. "Subcision: A Treatment for Cellulite." *International Journal of Dermatology.* 2000:539-544.

"How can I get rid of cellulite?" *Johns Hopkins Med Lett Health After 50.* February 2004; 15(12): 8.

Kaplan, Daile. *Albert Arthur Allen: Premier Nudes.* Santa Fe, New Mexico: Twin Palms Publishers, 2001.

Kelly, Katie. "Pinpoint Fat Relief?" *US News and World Report,* 10 March 2003, pg. 56.

Klein, William Arnold, ed. *Tissue Augmentation in Clinical Practice.* New York: Marcel Dekker, Inc., 1998.

Le Coz, Jacques, M.D. *Overview of Mesotherapy* prepared for International Society of Mesotherapie.

Lennon, Christine. "Is this the End for Cellulite?" *The New York Times,* 19 May 2005, pg. G3.

Lorenc, Z. Paul, M.D., F.A.C.S. and Hall, Trish. *A Little Work: Behind the Doors of a Park Avenue Plastic Surgeon.* New York: St. Martin's Press, 2004.

Lotti, T., M.D., Ghersetich, I., M.D., Grappone C., Ph.D., and Dini, G., Ph.D. "Proteoglycans in So-Called Cellulite." *International Journal of Dermatology.* May 1990: 272-274.

Suggested Reading *(Continued)*

Mashiah A., Berman V., Thole H.H., Rose S.S., Pasik S., Schwarz H., Ben-Hur H. "Estrogen and progesterone receptors in normal and varicose saphenous veins." *Cardiovasc Surg*. April 1999; 7(3): 327-31.

Matarasso, Alan, M.D. "Venous Thrombosis and Tight Underwear." *Arch. Intern. Med*. January 22, 1996; 156.

Matarasso, Alan, M.D., Pfeifer, Tracy M., M.D., and the Plastic Surgery Educational Foundation DATA Committee. "Mesotherapy for Body Contouring." *Plastic and Reconstructive Surgery*. April 15, 2005; Vol. 115, No. 5:1420-1423.

Mauriege, P., Galitzky, J., Berlan, M. and LaFontan, M. "Heterogeneous distribution of beta and alpha-2 adrenoceptor binding sites in human fat cells from various fat deposits: functional consequences." *European Journal of Clinical Investigation*. 1987; 17: 156-165.

Merlen J.F., Curri S.B. "Anatomico-pathological causes of cellulite." *J Mal Vasc*. 1984; 9 Suppl A: 53-4.

"Mesotherapy: Innovative French Technique to Eliminate Cellulite, Wrinkles, Pain, and Much More." *Ross and Marion Hauser's Caring Medical Newsletter*. May 2001: 1-4.

Mirrashed F., Sharp J.C., Krause V., Morgan J., Tomanek B. "Pilot study of dermal and subcutaneous fat structures by MRI in individuals who differ in gender, BMI, and cellulite grading." *Skin Res Technol*. August 2004; 10(3): 161-8.

Mori, Y., Kioka, E., Tokura, H. "Effects of pressure on the skin exerted by clothing on responses of urinary catecholamines and cortisol, heart rate and nocturnal urinary melatonin in humans." *Int. J. Biometeorol*. September 12, 2002; 47:1-5.

Nazarieff, Serge. *Early Erotic Photography*. Koln: Taschen GmbH., 2002.

Nurnberger, F. and Muller G. "So-Called Cellulite: An Invented Disease." *Journal of Dermatoloic Surgery and Oncology*. 4; 221-229.

Piérard, Gérald E., M.D., Ph.D., Nizet, J.L., M.D., and Piérard-Franchimont, Claudine, M.D., Ph.D. "Cellulite: From Standing Fat Herniation to Hypodermal Stretch Marks." The American *Journal of Dermatology*. 2000: 34-37.

Pierard-Franchimont C., Pierard G.E., Henry F., Vroome V., Cauwenbergh G. "A randomized, placebo-controlled trial of topical retinol in the treatment of cellulite." *Am J Clin Dermatol*. November-December 2000; 1(6): 369-74.

Querleux B., Cornillon C., Jolivet O., Bittoun J. "Anatomy and physiology of subcutaneous adipose tissue by in vivo magnetic resonance imaging and spectroscopy: relationships with sex and presence of cellulite." *Skin Res Technol*. May 2002; 8(2): 118-24.

Rao J., Paabo K.E., Goldman M.P. "A double-blinded randomized trial testing the tolerability and efficacy of a novel topical agent with and without occlusion for the treatment of cellulite: a study and review of the literature." *J Drugs Dermatol*. July-August 2004(4): 417-25.

Ribaudo, Charles A., M.D. and Formato, Anthony A., M.D. "Panty Girdle Syndrome." *New York State Journal of Medicine*. February 1, 1965; 456-457.

Rosenbaum M., Prieto V., Hellmer J., Boschmann M., Krueger J., Leibel R.L., Ship AG. "An exploratory investigation of the morphology and biochemistry of cellulite." *Plast Reconstr Surg*. June 1998; 101(7): 1934-9.

Rossi A.B., Vergnanini AL. "Cellulite: a review." *J Eur Acad Dermatol Venereol*. July 2000; 14(4): 251-62.

Scherwitz C., Braun-Falco O. "So-called cellulite." *J Dermatol Surg Oncol*. March 1978; 4(3): 230-4.

Scribner, Charles. *Rubens*. New York: Harry N. Abrams, Inc., 1989.

Singer, Sydney Ross, Grismaijer Soma. *Dressed to Kill*. Pahoa, Hawaii: ISCD Press, 2002.

Tostes R.C., Nigro D., Fortes Z.B., Carvalho M.H. "Effects of estrogen on the vascular system." *Braz J Med Biol Res*. September 2003; 36(9): 1143-58. Epub, August 19, 2003.

Wahrenberg, H.F. Lonnqvist, and P. Arner. 1989. "Mechanisms underlying regional differences in lipolysis in human adipose tissue." *J. Clin. Invest*. 84: 458-467.

Weihua Z., Andersson S., Cheng G., Simpson E.R., Warner M., Gustafsson J.A. "Update on estrogen signaling." *FEBS Lett*. July 3, 2003; 546(1): 17-24.

Winer, Susan, Wallis. Robert M.D. (preface). *Cellulite*. New York: Dell Publishing Company, 1975.

Mesotherapy Resources

ARIZONA
Dr. Christopher Breeden
Tucson, AZ
Ph: 520-940-8089

ARKANSAS
Dr. Jason C. Brandt
Eden Medical Spa
411 Union St.
Jonesboro, AR 72401
Ph: 870-931-3223
www.edenmedspa.com

CALIFORNIA
Dr. Donna Alderman
Hemwall Family Medical Centers
2915 Telegraph Ave., Ste. 301
Berkeley, CA 91208
Ph: 510-549-1700
1740 Broadview Dr.
Glendale, CA 91208
Ph: 818-957-3000

Dr. Mark Greenspan
4849 Van Nuys Blvd., Ste. 103
Sherman Oaks, CA 91403
Ph: 818-475-6100
Fx: 818-475-6188
markgspan@aol.com

Dr. Dwight Hiscox
Flash Laser Aesthetics
17401 Ventura Blvd., Ste. B-9
Encino, CA 91316
Ph: 818-205-1280
Fx: 828-205-1235
www.flashmeso.com
www.flashlaser.com

Dr. Lance Maki
Restoration Medicine
2123 Ygnacio Valley Road
Building K, Ste. 210
Walnut Creek, CA 94598
Ph: 925-933-MESO (6376)
www.restorationmedicine.com

Dr. Karl Norris
Beverly Hills Triangle
Medical Plaza
9735 Wilshire Blvd., Ste. 309
Beverly Hills, CA 90212
Ph: 310-859-8051
Fx: 310-274-4921
www.mesotherapy.com

Dr. Ron Rothenberg
Medical Education
Director, Bissoon Institute
of Mesotherapy
California HealthSpan Institute
320 Santa Fe Dr.
San Diego CA 92024
Ph: 760-635-1996
Ph: 800-943-3331
Fx: 760-635-1994
www.MDMesotherapy.com
www.eHealthSpan.com

FLORIDA
Dr. Joseph Averback
2865 PGA Blvd.
Palm Beach, FL 33410
Ph: 561-804-7500
Fx: 561-748-6778
www.pbgmesotherapy.com
md@pbgmesotherapy.com

Dr. Lionel Bissoon
President, Bissoon Institute
of Mesotherapy
Palm Beach
1411 North Flagler Dr., Ste. 4100
West Palm Beach, FL 33407
Ph: 561-838-4991
www.mesotherapy.com

Dr. Donna Dyer
433 SE Ocean Blvd., Ste. A
Stuart, FL 34994
Ph: 772-286-4045
Fx: 772-286-4051
idealdoc@earthlink.net
www.drdonnadyer.com

Joseph F. Greco, PhD. PAd
David M. Wall, M.D.
Cosmetic and Anti-Aging Solutions
3023 Eastland Blvd., Ste. 113
Clearwater, FL 33761
Ph: 727-791-3830
www.nosurgerysolutions.com

Dr. Jeffery A. Hunt
The Vein Center of Tampa Bay
3001 N. Rocky Point Drive East, Ste. 125
Tampa, FL 33607
Ph: 813-282-0223
Fx: 813-282-0190
www.veincentertampa.com

Dr. Enrique Monasterio
401 S. LeJeune Rd., 3rd Floor
Miami, FL 33134
Ph: 305-447-9111
Fx: 305 446-5708
www.medspamiami.com

Dr. Mercedes Montealegre
9872 Linebaugh Ave.
Tampa, FL 33626
Ph: 813-920-3500
Fx: 813-920-9011

Dr. G. Michael Nauert
A New You Laser Center
Clearwater, FL 33756
Ph: 727-442-6700
Fx: 727-442-2508

Dr. Sherri Pinsley
1325 S. Congress Ave., Ste. 207
Boyton Beach, FL 33426
Ph: 561-752- 5776

Dr. Jacqueline Redondo
10300 Sunset Dr., Ste. 282
Miami, FL 33173
Ph: 305-412-2800
Fx: 305-412-6045

Dr. Laura Rodriquez
233 Aragon Ave.
Coral Gables, FL 33134
Ph: 786-552-6800
Fx: 786-552-6801
www.Herenciasalonandspa.com

Mesotherapy Resources *(Continued)*

Dr. Dan Stein
Stein Medical Institute
2713 W. Virginia Ave.
Tampa, FL 33607
Ph: 813-873-9700
Fx: 813-873-9800

Dr. Manuel Suarez, F.A.C.C.P.
1435 W. 49 Place, Ste. 207
Hialeah, FL 33012
Ph: 305-556-8556
Fx: 305-556-6112
docrite@hotmail.com

GEORGIA
Dr. Lisa Merritt
International Medical Clinics
International Plaza, Ste. B4
5979 Buford Highway
Doraville, GA 30340
Ph: 678-547-0000
Fx: 678-547-0191
www.intimedicalclinics.come/home

ILLINOIS
Dr. Ross Hauser
715 Lake St., Ste. 600
Oak Park, IL 60301
Ph: 708-848-7789
Fx: 708-848-7763
www.caringmedical.com
info@caringmedical.com

Dr. Yakov Ryabor
Board Certified: Internal Medicine
Board Certified: Anti-aging Medicine
201 E. Strong Ave., Ste. 9
Wheeling, IL 60090
Ph: 847-419-1900
Fx: 847-419-1964

INDIANA
Dr. Lea Marlow
Marlow Laser Aesthetics
1201 East Spring St.
New Albany, IN 47150
Ph: 812-945-6142
www.DRMARLOW.com

LOUISIANA
Dr. Thomas Guillot, Jr.
**Faculty, Bissoon Institute
of Mesotherapy**
Plastic & Reconstructive Surgery
7777 Hennessy Blvd., Ste. 6001
Baton Rouge, LA 70808
Ph: 225-769-2955
Fx: 225-769-4908

MASSACHUSETTS
Dr. Laurent Delli-Bovi
Aesthetic Options
822 Boylston St., Ste. 109
Chestnut Hill, MA 02467
Ph: 617-277-0009
Fx: 617-277-3248

Kira Medspa,
North Andover main office:

Thomas Johnson, M.D., F.A.C.P.
Kenneth R. Dovidio, P.A.-C., M.H.P.
Susan Butterworth, R.N.C.S., N.P.
555 Turnpike St.
North Andover, MA 01845
Ph: 978-687-6373
www.KIRAMEDSPA.COM

Also offices in:
Kira Medspa Newburyport
The Professional Building
Forrester St.
Newburyport, MA 01950
Ph: 978-463-3760

MARYLAND
Caryl G. Mussenden, M.D., F.A.C.O.G.
Member of the American Academy
of Cosmetic Surgery
Gynecology and Liposuction
for Men & Women
9811 Greenbelt Rd., #104
Lanham, MD 20706
Ph: 301-552-1111
Fx: 301-552-9555

MICHIGAN
Dr. Salvatore Cavaliere
**Faculty, Bissoon Institute
of Mesotherapy**
1349 Rochester Road, Ste. 100
Rochester Hills, MI 48307
Ph: 248-651-5051
Fx: 248-651-5053

Also offices in:
Birmingham, MI 48150
Ph: 248-651-5051
Fx: 248-651-6053

Dr Charles Mok
Michigan Mesotherapy
8180 26 Mile Rd., Ste. 105
Shelby Township, MI, 48316
Ph: 586-992-8300
www.michiganmesotherapy.com

Dr. Gregory Shannon, M.B.A., F.A.C.E.T.
Advanced Health, Image
and Wellness Center
1650 Haslett Rd./P.O. Box 40
Haslett (Lansing), MI 48840-0040
Ph: 517-339-8900
Fx: 517-339-4230
www.shannonmd.com
greg@shannonmd.com
Affiliate MI locations: Brighton, Troy

NEVADA
Dr. Graham Simpson
Ageless-Zone
5050 Meadow Wood Mall Circle
Reno, NV 89502
Ph: 775-823-9665
www.agelesszone.com

NEW HAMPSHIRE
Thomas Johnson, M.D., F.A.C.P.
Kenneth R. Dovidio, P.A.-C., M.H.P.
Susan Butterworth, R.N.C.S., N.P.

Kira Medspa, Salem
Ph: 603-898-2695

Kira Medspa, Derry
Ph: 603-434-3810

Kira Medspa, Hampstead
Ph: 603-329-4294

Mesotherapy Resources *(Continued)*

NEW JERSEY

Dr. Mark James Bartiss
Institute for Complementary and
Alternative Medicine
24 Nautius Dr., Ste. 5
Manahawkin, NJ 08050
Ph: 609-978-9002

Dr. Lee Elber
Faculty, Bissoon Institute
of Mesotherapy
Mesotherapy Solutions of
New Jersey
100 W. Mt. Pleasant Ave.
Livingston, NJ 07039
Ph: 973-992-8111
Fx: 973-992-4145
www.mesosolutionsofnj.com

Dr. Anna D. Lee
1930 East Marlton Pike., Ste. L-63
Cherry Hill, NJ 08003
PH: 856-424-8236
Fx: 856-424-1150

Dr. Ed Magaziner
Mesotherapy Center of New Jersey
2186 Route 27, Ste. 2D
North Brunswick, NJ 08902
Ph: 732-297-5669
Fx: 732-297-5770

Dr. Sala Taha, F.A.C.S.
Vein Laser Center
550 Summit Ave., Ste. 203
Jersey City, NJ 07306
Ph: 201-795-9007
Fx: 201-659-0405
www.mesonj.com
www.vlcnj.com

NEW MEXICO

James E. Baum, D.O.
1850 Ols Pecos Trail, Ste. L
Santa Fe, NM 84505
Ph: 505-989-8647
Px: 505-983-6464
www.drjamesbaum.com
drbaum@comcast.net

NEW YORK

Dr. Lionel Bissoon
President, Bissoon Institute
of Mesotherapy
10 West 74th St., Ste. 1E
New York, NY 10023
Ph: 212-579-9136
Fx: 212-579-6917
www.mesotherapy.com

Dr. Denis F. Branson
7000 E. Genesee St. Bldg. E
Fayetteville, NY 13066
Ph: 315-446-8313
Fx: 315-446-5387
www.DrBranson.com
info@drbranson.com

Dr. Natalie Chen
Long Island, NY
Ph: 516-567-4764
hchen@optonline.net

Dr. Muneer Imam
295 Montauk Highway
Speonk, NY 11972
Ph: 361-878-0310
Fx: 361-878-0754
www.drimam.com
www.drimam@aol.com

Oz Garcia, Ph.D., Nutritionist
Personal Best, Inc.
10 West 74th St., Ste. 1G
New York, NY 10023
Ph: 212-362-5569

Dr. Harold Mermelstein
559 Gramatan Ave.
Mount Vernon, NY 10552
Ph: 914-667-2242
Fx: 914-667-8521

NORTH CAROLINA

Dr. Mitchell Bloom
The Center for Mind-Body Medicine
6518 Bryan Blvd., Ste. 100
Greensboro, NC 27409
Ph: 336-605-7077
Fx: 336-605-5577
www.mbmedicine.com

OHIO

David Garcia, D.O.
Roger Garcia, D.O.
Polaris Urgent Care Clinics
1120 Polaris Parkway, Ste. 100
Columbus, OH 43240
Ph: 614-847-1120

Dr. Diane McCormick
6011 Renaissance Place, #4
Toldeo, OH 43623
Ph: 419-885-5929
Fx: 419-824-6436

Dr. Mary Beth Mudd
New You Center for
Advanced Medical, L.L.C.
660 Cooper Road, Ste. 700
Westerville, OH 43081
Ph: 614-890-0365
Fx: 614-890-1677

OKLAHOMA

Dr. Martin R. Hullender, Jr.
304 South Park Ln.
Altus, OK 73521
Ph: 580-477-7356

PENNSYLVANIA

Dr. Marcia C. Dietrich
The Dietrich Medical Center
8 Church Ln.
Douglassville, PA 19518
Ph: 610-385-3022
Fx: 610-385-4446
drmarcia@aol.com

TEXAS

Ashley M. Classen, D.O.
The Institute of Age Management
and Aesthetic Medicine
Ph: 817-336-6461
1401 Henderson St.
Fort Worth, TX 76102
a.classen@iamrenewed.com
www.ageandaestheticmedicine.com

Mesotherapy Resources *(Continued)*

Dr. Gary Cox
Coastal Skin Care
2700 Citizens Plaza, Ste. 100
Victoria, TX 77901
Ph: 361-582-5770
800-475-4643

Dr. Mathew Schoen
610 Rainer Court
Highland Village, TX 75077
Ph: 972-727-2800

Dr. Jamie Vasquez
2929 Welborn St.
Dallas, TX 75219
Ph: 214-528-1083
Fx: 214-528-3252
Certified in Family Practice
www.vasquezclinic.com
jvasquez@drjvasquez.com

TENNESSEE

Dr. Laurie Baker
Southwind Medical Specialists
3725 Champion Hills Dr., St 2000
Memphis, TN 38125
Ph: 901-367-9001
Fx: 901-565-8787

Dr. Joyce Brown
Brentwood Medical Spa
Professional Medical
Group Affiliation
1177 Old Hickory Blvd., Ste. 101
P.O. Box 3044
Brentwood TN 37027-3044
Ph: 615-717-4400
www.anuemedicalspa.com

Dr. Michael F. Counce
Memphis OBGYN Association, PC
7900 Highway 64
Bartlett, TN 38133
Ph: 901-485-2247

Also offices in:
6215 Humphreys Blvd., Ste. 401
Memphis TN 38120
Ph: 901-485-2247

And:
7705 Poplar Ave. Bldg. B, Ste. 340
Germantown, TN 38138
Ph: 901-485-2247

Dr. Michael Posey
Memphis Internal Medicine
6005 Park Ave., Ste. 900B
Memphis, TN 38119
Ph: 901-684-1322
mposey@MIMMD.com

VIRGINIA

Dr. Denise E. Bruner,
Faculty, Bissoon Institute
of Mesotherapy
5015 Lee Highway, #201
Arlington, VA 22207
Ph: 703-558-4949

Dr. Harry Camper
L'Idee Aesthetics & Gynecology
1992 Medical Ave.
Harrisonburg, VA 22801
Ph: 540-437-1296

Lisa Harris, M.D.
1115 Independence Blvd., #118
Virginia Beach, VA 23455
Ph: 757-490-559
Fx: 757-464-3427
www.lisaharrismd.com
lharris@chasewellnesscenter.com

Dr. Reina M. Wilson
Leisa Brewer, R.N., B.S.N.
Rejuvisage, LLC
1830 Town Center Dr., Ste. 101
Reston, VA 20190
Ph: 703-303-1118
www.rejuvisage.com

AUSTRALIA

Dr. Julie Epstein, M.B.B.S., F.R.A.C.P.
Nicole Bell, L.N.
Mesotherapy Australia
www.mesotherapy.com.au
info@mesotherapy.com.au
Ph: 02 9327 5733 or
Ph: 1300 668 573
Outside Australia:
Ph: + 61 2 9327 5733

Leslie Fischer
Executive Director,
Bissoon Institute
of Mesotherapy
10 West 74th St., Ste. 1E
New York, NY 10023
Ph: 310-467-2301
Fx: 212-579-6917
www.mesotherapy.com

Index

Note: All page numbers in italic type indicate photos. If associated text occurs
    on the same page as a photo, the page number is not repeated.

Index *(Continued)*

Note: All page numbers in italic type indicate photos. If associated text occurs
    on the same page as a photo, the page number is not repeated.

Index *(Continued)*

Note: All page numbers in italic type indicate photos. If associated text occurs on the same page as a photo, the page number is not repeated.

Index (Continued)

_____

Note: All page numbers in italic type indicate photos. If associated text occurs
on the same page as a photo, the page number is not repeated.

Index (Continued)

Note: All page numbers in italic type indicate photos. If associated text occurs
    on the same page as a photo, the page number is not repeated.

Note: All page numbers in italic type indicate photos. If associated text occurs on the same page as a photo, the page number is not repeated.

Index *(Continued)*

Note: All page numbers in italic type indicate photos. If associated text occurs
    on the same page as a photo, the page number is not repeated.

Index (Continued)

Note: All page numbers in italic type indicate photos. If associated text occurs on the same page as a photo, the page number is not repeated.

Index *(Continued)*

Note: All page numbers in italic type indicate photos. If associated text occurs on the same page as a photo, the page number is not repeated.

The Standard of Excellence In

Mesotherapy Training

THE BISSOON INSTITUTE is now offering certification in the most sought after medical specialty today.

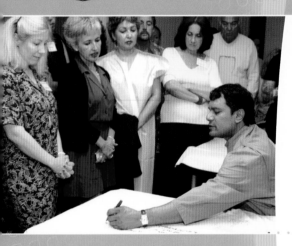

For four years Dr. Lionel Bissoon, the pioneer of Mesotherapy in the U.S., has been offering private training to the medical community. Due to overwhelming requests for this comprehensive, high-quality Mesotherapy training course, the Bissoon Institute will now offer open seminars on basic, intermediate, and advanced Mesotherapy procedures.

COURSE WORK INCLUDES:

- The Science of Mesotherapy
- Injection Techniques and Labs
- Stringcision™ and Surgical Subcision
- Presentations on medical and legal issues concerning pharmaceuticals and medical devices used in Mesotherapy
- Proper evaluation and treatment procedures for Cellulite, Overweight Patients and Spot Reduction
- Sterile techniques
- Evaluation of Thyroid with new parameters
- The basics of starting a successful Mesotherapy practice

"The course was head and shoulders above the rest. It was well organized, informative, educational, interesting and scientifically sound. Any physician who arrived to your course with no knowledge could start practicing SAFELY and immediately upon its completion."

Jacqueline Redondo, M.D., Miami, Florida

"It was probably one of the best courses I have attended during my medical career."

Helen Donatelli M.D., Miami, Florida

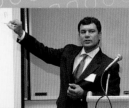

Lionel Bissoon, D.O., is widely acclaimed for having brought Mesotherapy to the United States in the late 1990s. The success of his practice has paved the way for others to administer Mesotherapy. Nearly all certified Mesotherapists in the United States utilize the techniques pioneered by Dr. Bissoon. He has been featured on *ABC's 20/20*, *CBS's 48 Hours*, *U.S. News & WORLD REPORT*, *People Magazine*, *Vogue* and others as the premier expert on Mesotherapy in the United States.

To sign up please visit www.mesotherapy.com or call (310) 467-2301

THE CELLULITE CURE™

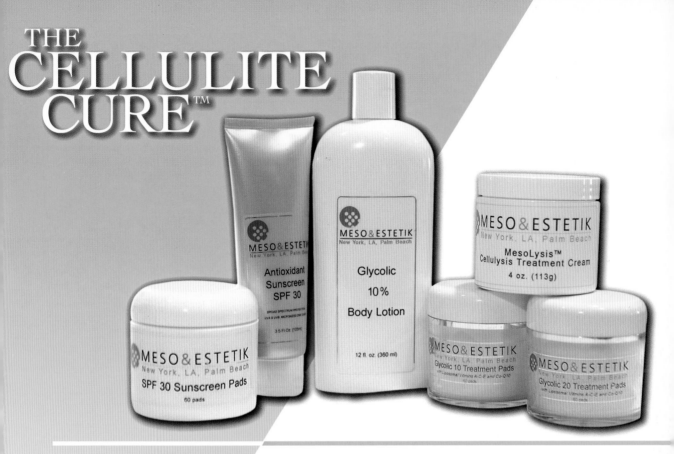

PRODUCTS

Cellulite Cream: MesoLysis™

Developed by Dr. Bissoon, this intense cream is formulated to help minimize the appearance of cellulite and increase the skin's hydration and elasticity while visibly improving and refining skin tone and texture.

Glycolic Treatment Pads

Glycolic acid treatment pads gently exfoliate, moisturize and assist in the removal of oils and residue on the skin while delivering to the skin toning and astringent benefits. *Available in a 10% glycolic recommended for the face and body.*

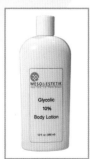

Glycolic 10% Body Lotion

Our lotion is cosmetically elegant and has been specially formulated to help achieve softer, smoother skin texture and tone. This light, quick absorbing lotion contains Vitamin E, Vitamin A and Vitamin C to condition the skin and assist in minimizing free-radical-induced skin damage.

Available at www.cellulitecure.com

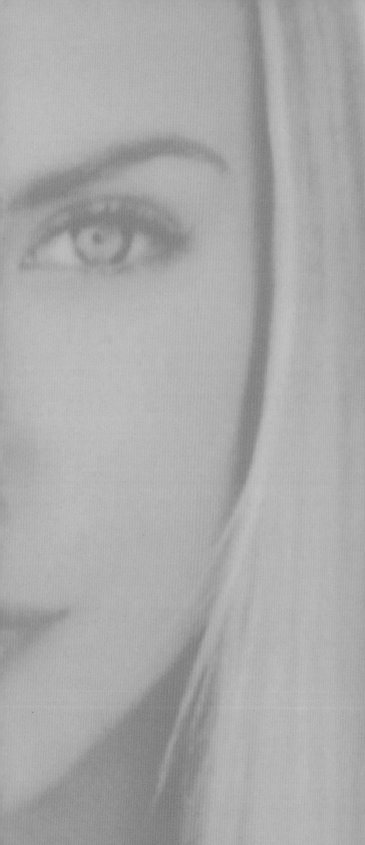

"If you are looking to create a successful medical spa you definitely need the guidance, knowledge, and expertise of Cheryl Whitman and her team of experts. From beginning to end, Cheryl is the greatest resource for creating the most successful and up to date medi spa."

Dr Lionel Bissoon
Pres. Bissoon Institute of Mesotherapy

"Cheryl has an amazing ability to combine business knowledge, marketing expertise and operational know-how with other aspects of medical and aesthetic treatments. She seems to know what will be hot before it is! She has been an invaluable asset in setting up the aesthetic treatments and office structure of our new comprehensive medical spa and cosmetic surgery center. She is the one consultant we could not have done without."

Julio Gallo, MD, FACS
The MIAMI Institute for
Age Management & Intervention
Located at the Four Seasons MIAMI

"Her expertise and the input on the many aspects of a spa business can be an invaluable resource for any medical professional "flirting" with the spa industry."

Hannalore R. Leavy
Executive Director, The Day Spa Association
& The International Medical Spa Association

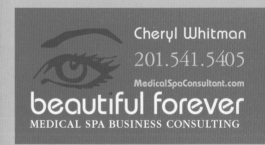

Cheryl Whitman
201.541.5405
MedicalSpaConsultant.com

beautiful forever
MEDICAL SPA BUSINESS CONSULTING

it's time to start our
beautiful relationship

Dr. Sears
ZONECafe

The Omega Zone Dietary Program

Most chronic disease like heart disease, diabetes, Alzheimer's—and aging itself—is caused by "Silent Inflammation."

Beauty in the skin is related to this same phenomena. Dr. Sears Omega Zone Dietary Program can greatly assist the Mesotherapy practitioner, when added to a total lifestyle approach. Living life in the Zone is achieved by "letting food be your ultimate medicine."

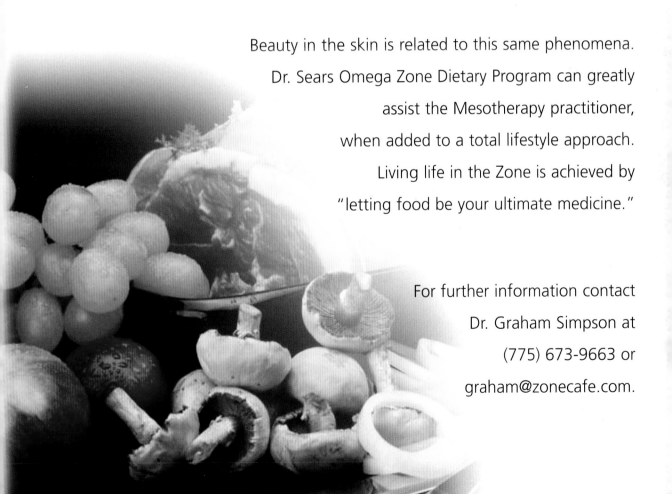

For further information contact Dr. Graham Simpson at (775) 673-9663 or graham@zonecafe.com.